Shotokan Karate Leadership School®

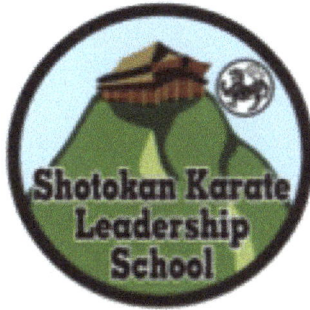

We grow leaders

Shoka Leader Handbook

Shoka Leader Handbook

Table of Contents

Introduction 5
   Welcome Letter...5
   Our Great Story...6
   The Black Belt Shoka Leader Program 7
   Tiger's Great Journey 7
   Our Great Houses...10
   Patches...10
   Points...11
   Your Instructors...12

Spirit and Mind 14
   Your Training..14
   Critical Martial Arts Lessons...16
   Our Guiding Principles:..19
       GF's 5 Rules...19
       Dojo Creed...20
       Niju Kun...21
       12 Shoka Traits..27
   Good Manners – Your First Line of Self Defense................28
   Rules and Procedures...30
   Class Commands..31
   Uniform..32
   Community Service 33

The Shoka Way of Leadership 34
   Why Shotokan Karate Leadership School 34
   Setting Goals..34
   The 4 Levels...36
   Teamwork...37
   Student Leaders..37
   Student Instructors...38
   How We Train Leaders 39
   The School...39
   Community Leadership 39

Shotokan Karate **40**
    Warm up Exercises..40
    Basic Stretches...43
    Basics/Kihon..44
    Sparring/Kumite...55
    Kata/Forms..59
        Heian Shodan..59
        Heian Nidan..62
        Heian Sandan..65
        Heian Yondan..67
        Heian Godan..69
        Tekki Shodan...71
        Advanced Katas...73
    Conditioning Exercises..74

Appendix **76**
    Japanese Terminology...76
    Ranking System...78
    Personal Record of Achievement......................................79

For Rank Requirements see your SKLS Workbook

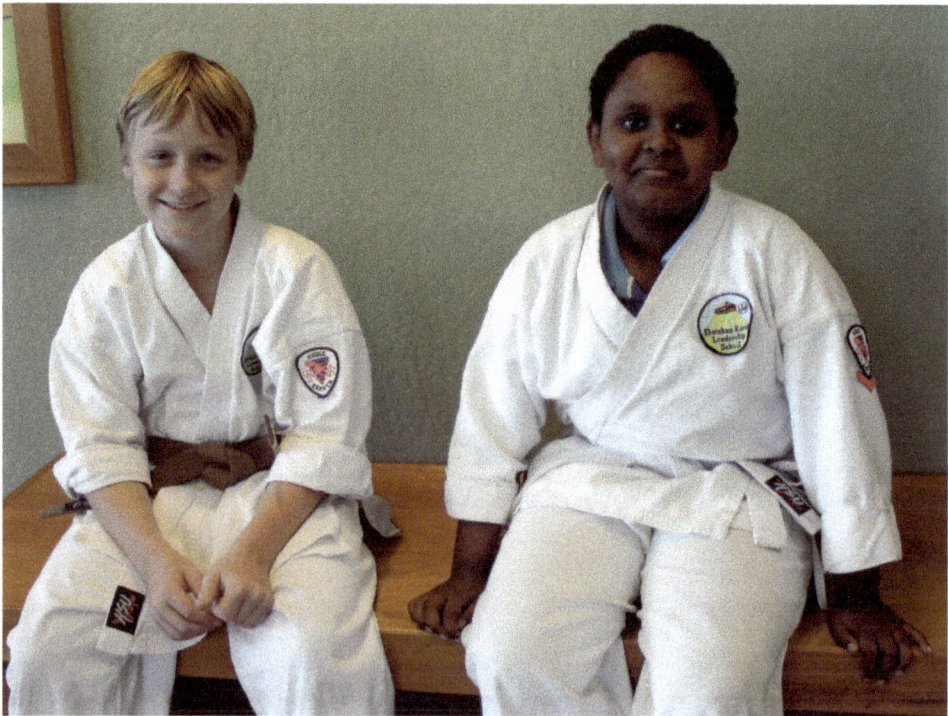

Introduction

From the Founder of Shotokan Karate Leadership School®

To You, A New SKLS Student;

If you want to become a LEADER, this letter is for you. You are facing a world that is getting more and more competitive every day, and if you want to do well, which I'm sure you do, you need to prepare; but what is the best preparation?

I believe you need to start by becoming the best possible version of yourself. This means developing character traits such as courage, courtesy, integrity, humility, self-control, trust, endeavor, responsibility, cooperation, justice, compassion and creativity. You will be establishing and enhancing these traits as you learn to kick, punch, and defend yourself against physical threats, because defending yourself in the 21st century is not about fighting evil-doers on a day-to-day basis, but taking on challenges that test the strength of your character.

Don't think for a moment this will be easy, because it won't. It is natural for you to not want to change. All you know is what you knew up until now, and changes can cause an upset as you figure out how to adjust. You must recognize that you need to change in order to become the person you want to be and have the good life you want to have.

Where do you start? Teach yourself to look at the world around you and see the problems that exist. Then, encourage yourself to find a solution to those problems. If the first solution you devise doesn't work, encourage yourself to create another one, and if that doesn't work, create another one. Before the light bulb was created, humans spent a good part of their lives in darkness. There were candles and other means to create light, but they were severely limited. Thomas Edison tried 1,000 times to solve the problem of lighting the darkness before he created the light bulb. Teach yourself not to give up. Teach yourself to persist. Listen for your life calling. Become a leader instead of settling for being a follower.

Everywhere you look there are problems, problems that need capable, intelligent leaders to solve them. That leader could be you. In addition to this course being about the fundamentals of self-defense, it is also a call to action. It's a call for you to awaken the extraordinary leader in yourself, and it's a call for you to act.

The question is, will you answer this call and let us help you become the person you are meant to be? I sincerely hope you will, and I look forward to having you as a leadership student.

Marty Callahan
Founder, CEO, 7th Degree Black Belt

Our Great Story – Shotokan Karate

As you begin your study of karate, you might be confused by the many different styles and philosophies you may have heard about. Karate is an Asian art of self-defense based on the proper use of the mind, body, and spirit. Its history is said to date back over 2,000 years, involving developments in India, China, Korea, and other countries.

Karate is an empty-handed system of self-defense that demands great discipline, and in return, gives practitioners enormous energy, confidence, and freedom. It is an art that was designed thousands of years ago by common people to protect themselves during times of war and to train leaders during times of peace. The creators of this art knew that the martial skills that prepared a warrior to face danger, lead the charge to battle, and outmaneuver a superior foe applied to leadership as well.

The early karate practitioners not only developed techniques and strategies for defense but also a set of ideals, principles, and organizational structures that provided security and a means to create a better future. The principles of character, sincerity, effort, etiquette and self-control guided their lives and made them even more valuable as leaders of their communities.

Gichin Funakoshi

Karate was introduced to Japan from Okinawa in 1922, when Master Gichin Funakoshi presented a demonstration in Tokyo. Karate in Okinawa had two primary schools; the *Shorei* school, primarily for large, powerful people that was characterized by forceful breathing and short, hard movements. The *Shorin* school was primarily for small, lighter people, and was characterized by sharp, fast, and long movements. Funakoshi combined the techniques of both schools into what he considered an all-inclusive style. Master Funakoshi never named his approach to karate, but his students called it *Shotokan*. Funakoshi was a poet and his pen name was *Shoto. Kan* means house, or building. Thus, we have the translation of *Shotokan*, or *"House of Funakoshi"*.

Shotokan karate stands out because of its founder, Gichin Funakoshi. As a school teacher in rural Okinawa, Funakoshi dreamed of karate being practiced around the world and dedicated his life to making this happen. Before him, karate was practiced in secret, with its principles, techniques, and spiritual essence passed down from teacher to student by word of mouth only. In the pursuit of his dream, Funakoshi organized karate into a coherent written system, establishing an organization and instructor training program that spread karate around the world.

Where others taught martial arts with an emphasis on fighting, Funakoshi emphasized karate's spiritual essence and refinement of character. Having been a schoolteacher, scholar of Chinese classics, and a calligrapher and poet, Funakoshi encouraged study and the practice of more genteel arts to balance karate. His strength of character drew people to him, led them to fulfill his mission, and energized them to take action against injustice.

Marty Callahan

Early in his training, the SKLS founder recognized karate's enormous potential to transform ordinary people into leaders. His attention has remained on awakening leaders. Marty Callahan has spent his life understanding and improving the lives of students both young and old. His passion for karate and leadership led to the founding of Shotokan Karate Leadership School® in Santa Rosa, California in 1981. His dream is to awaken the extraordinary leader in everyone, starting with his students. He has inspired, coached, supported, and trained over 10,000 students in over 30,000 classes. Hundreds of his students have gone on to become leaders in their chosen fields due to his engaging, student-centered approach to teaching.

The Black Belt Shoka Leader Program

The Black Belt Shoka Leader Program lays out a four-year path to become a black belt. It may take more or less time, depending on your age and how much you practice, but the average person achieves their black belt target date in four years. There are also character goals you must reach to achieve your black belt. In your first year, you strive to become an Independently Motivated Self-Starter. In your second year you will become a Productive Team Member. In your third year, you become a Result-Oriented Team Leader; and in your fourth year you will become a Humble Servant Leader of People.

Tiger's Great Journey

You've may have heard about or own a book that our school wrote; *Tiger's Great Journey* is an adventure story for youth who want to make the world a better place.   It is about a boy named Tiger who saw other kids being bullied and it left him feeling scared, helpless and angry. He wanted to do something about it, so he came into our school. After talking with one of our instructors, he decided that he would become a black belt. Then, he had a dream. In his dream he met a famous karate master, Gichin Funakoshi, and after talking with him decided that he would take a great journey to the top of Ryoku Mountain where he would take his black belt test in the Temple of the Clouds. But this would not be an easy journey – it would be one of the most difficult things Tiger ever did in his young life. To help him on his way Master Funakoshi presented Tiger with *The Book of the Empty Mind*. His friend, Blake, accompanies him on this character-building journey. Together they overcome obstacles and learn important life lessons.

Every student who enters our school and makes the decision to become a black belt is on their own Great Journey. Whether you are young or old this Great Journey will awaken the extraordinary leader in you. The leader who can dream, think, tell his or her story, and lead.

The Book of the Empty Mind

Another important part of SKLS training is introduced in *Tiger's Great Journey*, The Book of the Empty Mind journal. In the story, Gichin Funakoshi meets Tiger on the beach and gives him The Book of the Empty Mind. The book is empty because Tiger is supposed to fill it with his experiences as he learns more about karate and himself. You will be expected to fill your very own Book of the Empty Mind as you progress through the belt ranks. It's important to document your struggles and victories so you can understand your shortcomings and strengths and use them to help others on their journey to becoming a black belt.

Great Journey Map

The Great Journey Map draws your eye almost as soon as you step into a Shotokan Karate Leadership School®. It is based on Tiger's journey to the Temple of the Clouds, and allows you to see your progress on your way to black belt. You will have a piece on the map that represents you and your Great Journey. Talk with your school leaders about what you need to do to make this happen.

Tiger, in his Great Journey to the Temple of the Clouds, had to overcome 12 major challenges. These challenges developed in him the 12 Shoka Leadership traits of courage, courtesy, integrity, humility, self-control, trust, endeavor, responsibility, cooperation, justice, compassion and creativity. These 12 challenges and leadership traits are represented on the Great Journey Map with symbols. Your challenge is to find those symbols and relate them with to the 12 Shoka Leadership traits.

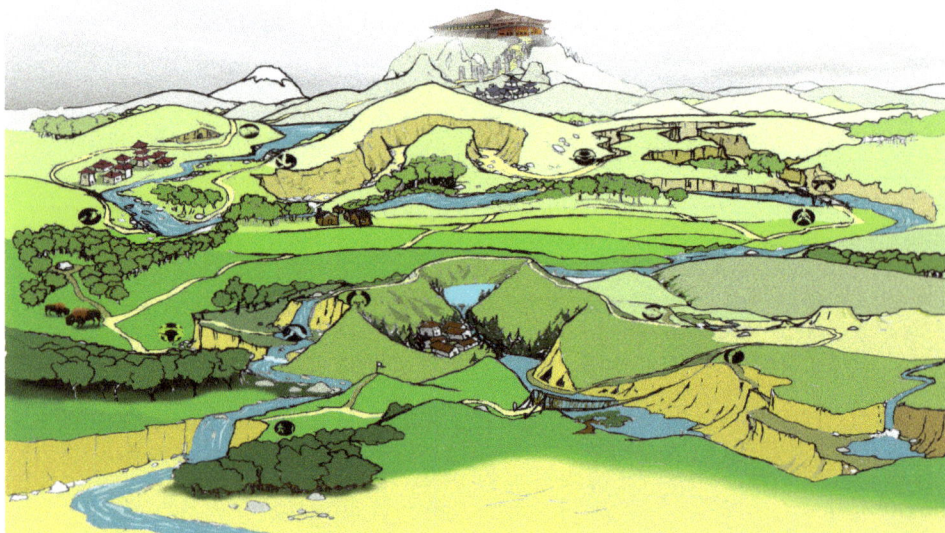

Your Workbook/Binder

You will receive a packet at the beginning of every month. The packet will be full of information on the curriculum topic for the month and how you can apply it in everyday life. You will have assignments every week to read a story or do a project. Sometimes you will need your parents' help, but you are the one who is becoming a black belt so you must take responsibility for doing the reading and completing the assignments and projects. There will be a written exam on the curriculum material at the end of each two-month period, so put the packet material in your BBSL binder. This will help you keep track of them and you can look back at past month's material.

Additional Reading Materials

You will have reading assignments from various sources included in your monthly packet, but you may also have reading assignments from any one of these world-changing leaders and authors:

Anthony Robbins	Zig Ziglar	Pres. Ronald Reagan
Gen. Norman Schwarzkopf	Gen. Colin Powell	Tim Cook
Brian Tracy	Jim Rohn	Dr. Dennis Watley
Warren Buffett	John C. Maxwell	Nido Qubein
Steve Jobs	Seth Godin	Dr. Shad Helmstetter
Gen. Martin Dempsey	Gichin Funakoshi	Joe Hyams
Dr. Terrance Webster-Doyle	Stephen Covey	Chuck Norris
Larry Donnithorn	Lee Milteer	Marty Callahan
Sun Tsu	Miyamoto Musashi	C. W. Nicol
Masatoshi Nakayama	Peter Urban	David Schwartz
Norman Vincent Peale	Maxwell Maltz	Dale Carnegie
Napoleon Hill	Peter Drucker	Clayton Christensen
Eliyahu Goldratt	Michael E. Gerber	Emmentt C. Murphy
Mark A. Murphy	Jeff Cannon	Max De Pree
Lt. Comdr. Jon Cannon	Kerry Patterson	Joseph Grenny
Ron McMillian	Al Switzler	James C. Collins
Jerry I. Porras	Catherine Ponder	Shakti Gawain
Benjamin Franklin	Robert T. Kiyosaki	J. Krishnamurti
Deepak Chopra	Muhammad Yunus	Roger Fisher
William Ury	Thomas J. Peters	Robert Cialdini
Robert H. Waterman Jr.	Richard Marchinko	Robert Cooper
Yamamoto Tsunetomo	Eugen Herrigel	Randall G. Hassell
Takuan Soho	Robert M. Pirsig	Stan Schmidt
Herman Kauz	Lao Tzu	Dan Carrison
Rod Walsh		

Our Great Houses

There are four houses to choose from when you enter the Black Belt Shoka Leader Program. The first is **House Terra**, for grounded people who like to make plans and are not easily disturbed. **House Kraken** is for people who go with the flow and want to make sure that everyone is happy. **House Fire Dragon** is for quick-tempered and strong-willed people. **House Sora** is for those who like to analyze and think things through. We're born with one or two of these qualities being more dominant than the others. In choosing a house you will want to choose the one that best describes you. The benefit of this is that you can learn about yourself and then learn about other people and what they're like. This knowledge will make engaging with others easier. Over time you will develop these and other qualities in yourself and be able to bring them out as situations demand. When you can do this, you will be said to be in the void, or the state of nothingness. If you'd like more information about this see the Book of Five Rings, by Miyamoto Musashi.

Patches

When you first joined Shotokan Karate Leadership School® you are fitted with a uniform. When you join the Black Belt Shoka Leader Program you will receive a school patch. The school patch is place on your uniform on the left side of your chest. When you choose a house you will receive a house patch, which is placed on your left shoulder below the seam. As you develop your leadership skills and take on various leadership roles you will receive other patches that will help students identify you. For more information about these leadership roles see the paragraph titled 'Student Leaders' in 'The Shoka Way of Leadership' section of this handbook.

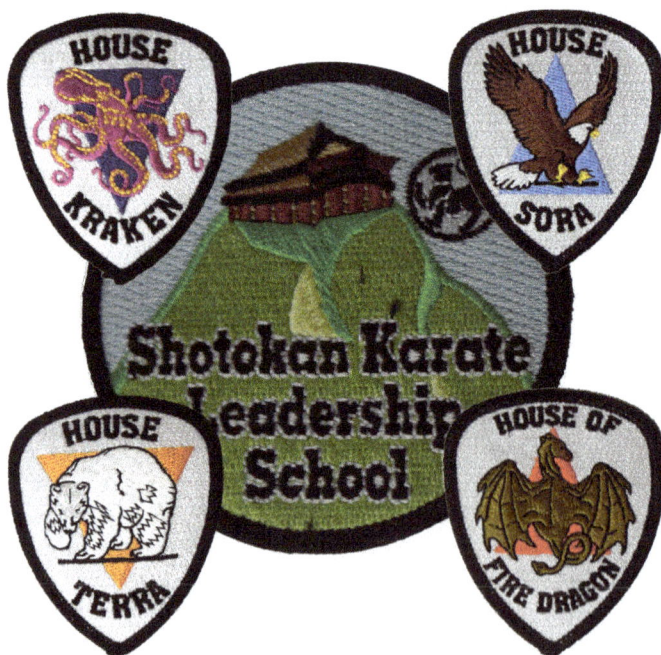

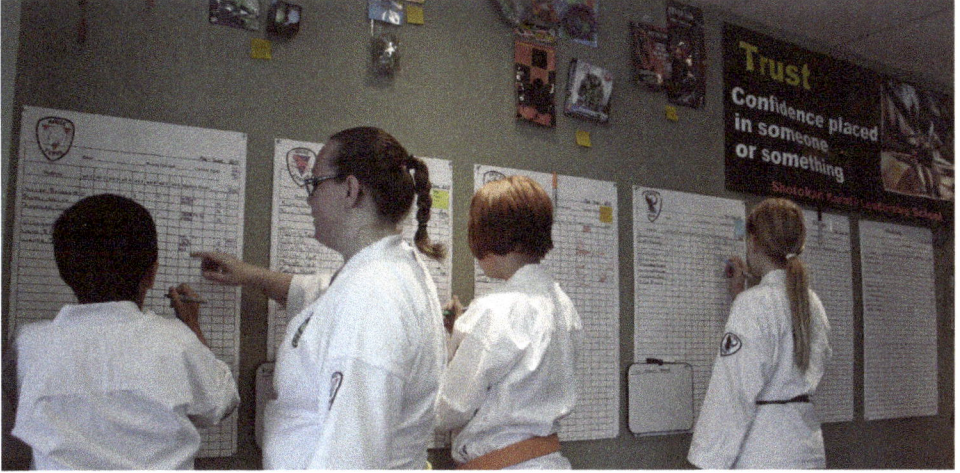

Points

A fun part of being in a house is that you get to earn points, which can be traded in for small prizes. And you get to earn points for your house, which can be traded in for fun activities such as a trip to the beach, roller skating, a movie night, a sleep over, pizza party, etc. You will keep an account of your points on your house's tracking sheet on the wall. Each time you come to class and apply yourself to your training you will receive two points and your house will receive one point.

Your Instructors

Your instructor is the key to this training process. He or she will provide you with the inspiration, education, training, coaching, and support you'll need. They have worked hard to get where they are, and, in a sense, he or she represents the highest values of martial arts training. They will show you how to succeed in every circumstance, and the lessons you learn will stay with you your whole life. Your sensei is committed to training you, and in return, you must commit yourself to practicing everything you learn. Your relationship with him or her is important, so pay attention to what they tell you.

Always address your instructor as 'Sensei.' This term is one of respect. The literal meaning of *sensei* is "one who has gone before," implying that your teacher has already succeeded at what you are about to attempt and can show you the proper way to do it. This prevents you from repeating the mistakes others have made in the past. Mistakes are an important part of learning and you'll make plenty of your own, but learning from the mistakes of others is just as important.

Say hello and goodbye to your instructor, both when you come to class and when you leave. This shows respect and teaches you to communicate with authority figures in your life. It is important to be considerate of your instructor's time, though. If they are caught up in a conversation, do not interrupt them to say goodbye. Instead, wave at them after you bow out. If they don't see you, it's perfectly fine.

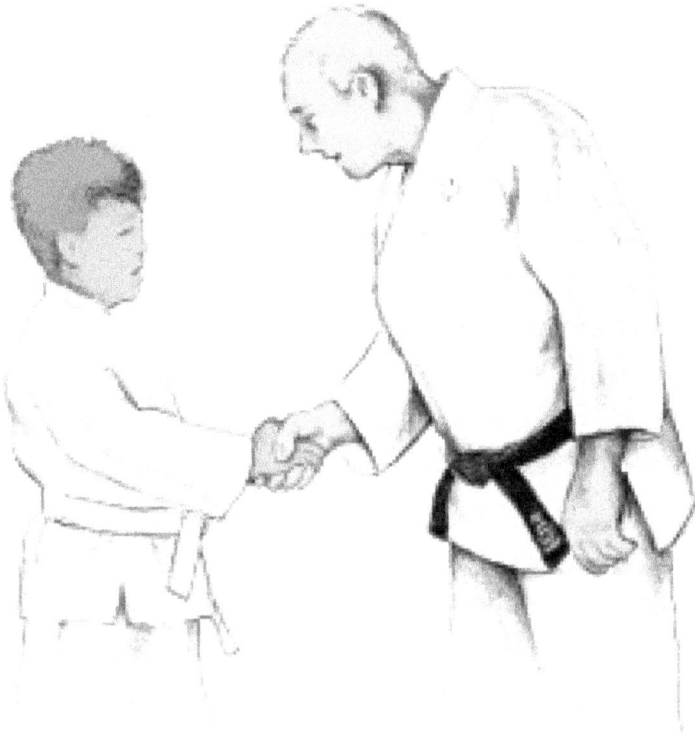

There are different levels of Instructors in Shotokan Karate Leadership School®:

Instructor: An Instructor is qualified to teach all levels and programs. The position is for an adult, with a minimum of 1st dan Black Belt. This position reports to the Senior Instructor.

An Instructor is a member of the School Board of Review and the Instructional Board. An Instructor wears the Instructor Patch on their left shoulder as well as two red chevrons below it. Instructors will line up slightly back and to the right of the Senior Instructor.

Senior Instructor: A Senior Instructor is qualified to oversee all Instructors. This position is for an adult who has earned 2nd dan Black Belt. A Senior Instructor reports to the Chief Instructor.

Senior Instructors are members of the School Board of Review, the Instructional Board, the Board of Examiners, and are Advisers to the Student Leaders Council. When lining up, the Senior Instructors stand slightly back and to the right of the Chief Instructor. They will wear a Senior Instructor bar above the Instructor Patch that sits above two red chevrons.

Chief Instructor: The Chief Instructor is qualified to oversee the instructional program. This position is for an adult who as achieved a minimum of 3rd dan Black Belt and reports to the Owner, Manager, or CEO of the school. Even though there may be more than one instructor in a school over the rank of 3rd dan, there is only one Chief Instructor of a school.

The Chief Instructor's role is to chair the School Board of Review, the Instructional Board and the Board of Examiners. The Chief Instructor lines up front and center on the training floor and wears the Chief Instructor bar above the Instructor Patch and two red chevrons.

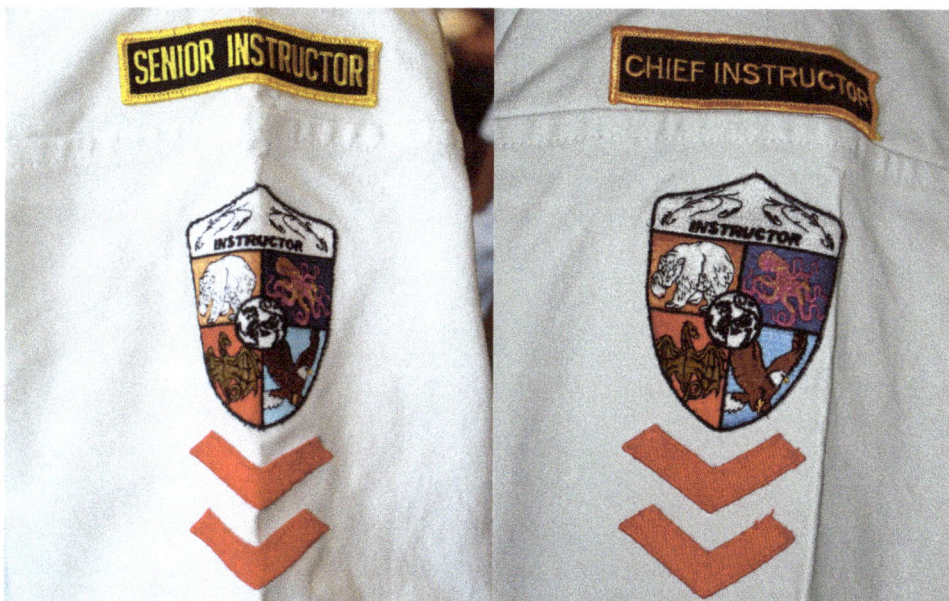

Spirit and Mind

Your Training

To Infinity and Beyond

If you always think of yourself as a beginner, then you will remain humble about your abilities. You will also have infinitely more potential to succeed when you are open about your flaws. You will also want to develop the mentality of staying with something forever. If you have this mental state, your ability to succeed will increase exponentially. If you believe this, you will be a better student and a better person. Accepting and embracing a certain part of your life as if it is there to stay will be crucial to your growth as a leader.

Your Black Belt Target Date

When you joined the Black Belt Shoka Leader Program, you made a commitment to becoming a black belt. You may or may not have set a black belt target date right away. If you did not, you can set one in any leadership class or make an appointment with an instructor to discuss it. It typically takes about four years to become a black belt, but it can be done in less time if you dedicate yourself to regular practice and keep good attendance. Set a reasonable goal, and you can adjust it if you need. After you reach 1st kyu brown belt, make an appointment with your instructor to talk about your Black Belt Target Date. He or she will set up a time for you to take private lessons in preparation for your black belt test. Shotokan Karate Leadership School® holds black belt tests twice a year, in June and December.

Pause if you need to… But never stop

It's important to take a break if you are exhausted, but it is also important to come back to what you were doing. Don't leave your homework half-finished or your jobs at home undone. Take a short break so you can approach it in a fresh light. You may need to take a break from karate at some point, whether for health reasons, or schoolwork. Don't quit, though. You made a commitment to become a black belt, and you need to keep your promise to yourself. You can do anything you set your mind to.

Practice

It is very important that you spend at least ten minutes every day stretching and training. There is a reason practicing is required in order for you to promote. If you practice outside of the school, you will be able to advance faster and understand karate better. It's important to try things on your own. It's good that you're learning from your instructor, but part of your training is about being an *independently motivated self-starter*. You are not supposed to be dependent on your teacher at school to make sure you do your homework. If you don't do your homework, you will fail the class. Karate works much the same way. If you don't practice, you will have a hard time advancing, especially as you move up in the ranks.

Plan to practice your kata at least once a day. If you regularly set time aside to practice, you can reach your goals faster. If you stretch everyday, you will become more flexible. Practicing your kata outside of class can help you understand the kata and perfect it faster. Practice makes permanent, so practice as often as you can. It doesn't have to be a huge amount of time or even the best practice ever. Often, you will hit plateaus and feel like you've hit a giant wall, but the practice will pay off, and you will see the results you want if you keep pushing. Endeavor and persist, even when it feels like you mess up a certain move every time you practice your kata. If you keep doing the move over and over again, you will get it right. Remember that karate isn't meant to be easy, it's meant to make you into a better person.

The Spirit of Giving

You've probably heard your parents talk about the spirit of giving around Christmas, but giving is important all the time. You should give all your attention and concentration to the one thing you are doing at the moment. If you're washing dishes, you should wash the dishes the best you know how. If you're doing schoolwork, do it really well. If you're practicing karate, pay attention to your instructor and not to your classmates. You should give your all when it comes to karate. Don't give your all to fooling around when you're supposed to be practicing kata. It is important to have fun, but there is a time and place to have fun. You can jump pads and do obstacle courses after you work hard.

It is also important to give your help to others. If you have a leadership position at the school, do your best. Give encouragement and direction to as many people as possible. If you have a hard time being patient with your siblings or remembering to take time to tell your mom you love her, give them the gift of your time or an "I love you." It's better to give than to take. When you give, you receive the gratification of making someone else happy, so give someone a hug or a smile today. You can make someone's day brighter.

Beyond Black Belt

Karate is still important even after you get your black belt. The life lessons you have learned will stay with you for the rest of your life, and your training will come back to you when you need to defend yourself. When you've earned your first-degree black belt you are considered to have mastered the basics but that's only the starting point. First-degree black belt is often said to be an advanced beginner. Karate is something you can practice your whole life. Master Funakoshi began his training at a very young age. According to some historians he may have started as young as 4 years old. And he continued to practice up until about a week before he died at 90 years old. That means he practiced for about 85 years. All the while he felt that he was still learning. Push yourself to higher levels of excellence and self-discovery. Shotokan Karate training could be a lifelong pursuit if you let it.

Critical Martial Arts Lessons

Re-establish Peace: The True Purpose of War and Self-defense

War was created to re-establish peace, even though it sounds contradictory. Self-defense is a natural human response to danger. It is often called your fight or flight mechanism, and you can learn to control and fine-tune it. Its purpose is also to neutralize the threat and restore the previously existing peace. It is not to humiliate your attacker or cause them more pain than necessary. Be careful to always keep this in mind, with whatever you do.

Battles are Won by Thinking...Not by Fighting

Behind all the foot soldiers and cavalry are the generals directing attacks and retreats. Every battle won requires a general who thought of a plan to defeat their enemy. Some of the most brilliant minds in history were generals in an army. Just as wars are won by thinking, so are the everyday battles you fight. Maybe you lost your favorite shirt, and your plan to find it is to clean your room. If a bully attacks you, think of what you can do to stop them from hurting you without causing them any damage. Get an adult and tell them about what happened. Every problem you face can be solved by thinking. Sometimes it will take a little more thinking than other problems would, but don't give up.

Violence is Seldom the Answer

But when it is, it's the only answer. Use your words to neutralize the situation. Talk your way out of everything you can. Often, people who are angry with you will listen to what you have to say. However, there are people who won't listen to reason or flattery, and believe that hurting you is the best way to appease their anger. Violence is needed to stop this individual from hurting or killing you. You have to cause them some pain in order for them to leave you alone.

The True Meaning of the Martial Arts

Many people have used the martial arts to gain wealth and power over others, but this is not its true purpose. The true intent of martial arts is to stop conflict, creating peace.

Conflict begins in the mind and expresses itself through behavior. Thoughts about a subject develop in the mind until they become beliefs. When a belief is formed, the person who holds this belief will act immediately on it without any further thought. If a person of one belief encounters a person that holds a different belief on the same subject, then the conditions are ripe for conflict. Fighting with someone who thinks differently than you is senseless. You will be fighting with everyone you encounter. Who wants to live like that? Similarly, you can have conflicting beliefs in your own mind. Beating yourself up over this is a waste of time. You would do far better to pause and recognize the fact that you have different beliefs than another person and you should respect them both.

Karate is a martial art that uses countless repetitions of techniques demanding a concentrated mental focus. This focus is to empty the mind of negative thoughts and emotions that are the root of conflict. The word 'karate,' implies this. It is actually two words, '*kara*' and '*te*,' meaning "empty hand," and by extension, "empty mind." Each technique, when properly executed, is stopped just before completion, allowing the student the time to consider the action before finishing it.

But stopping your technique is not enough. If you find yourself in conflict with another person, you have a duty to try to understand how they think and act. To do this, you must watch and listen carefully without fear. Once you have achieved understanding of the other person, the way is clear for them to understand you and for a peaceful solution to be found. A true martial artist is someone who stops their own internal conflict, making him or herself a more peaceful person, and interacting with others in a calmer way.

An excellent application of these principles is found in the story of...

The Wooden Rooster

Many years ago there lived an Emperor who had a magnificent rooster. This rooster was young, strong, amazingly quick, and strikingly handsome; the envy of the chicken yard.

The Emperor decided that he wanted to test his rooster in a fight with other roosters, according to the customs of those days. So the Emperor sent out a message to the best rooster trainer in the land, inviting him to come to his palace.

When the trainer arrived, the Emperor asked him if he would train his rooster. The trainer agreed, but only on one condition. The Emperor could only make the rooster fight when the trainer said he was ready, and not before. The Emperor consented, and the trainer departed with the prize rooster.

After some time had passed, the Emperor sent a message to the trainer, inquiring if his rooster was ready to fight. The trainer replied with a simple message: The rooster was not ready, and he needed more training. So the Emperor waited impatiently. After another month or two, he was eager to start his rooster in a fight. He sent another message to the trainer asking if his rooster was ready. The trainer again responded with a firm no, the rooster needed more training. He politely asked the Emperor to be patient and wait. But after another period of time, the Emperor couldn't bear waiting any longer. He again sent a message to the trainer, demanding to know if his rooster was ready. This time, the trainer replied that his rooster was ready.

The Emperor sent a servant to retrieve his rooster so he could take him to a kingdom-wide rooster fight, where only the best fighting roosters in the kingdom were gathering. The Emperor placed his rooster in the ring and sat down, expectant of a good show. Instead of attacking the other roosters, however, the Emperor's rooster walked to the center of the ring and stood perfectly still. He was so still and quiet, he appeared to be wooden.

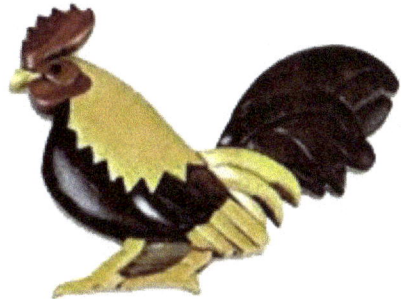

The other roosters glanced at the Emperor's rooster, but his stillness confused them. They weren't afraid of him and they didn't attack him. After a bit, the stillness and peacefulness of the Emperor's rooster began to have a calming effect on the other roosters. Deep inside, at their very core, the roosters preferred peace to war. They had been trained to fight each other against their nature. One by one, their movements slowed, and after only a few minutes, all fighting ceased.

The Emperor's rooster was declared the winner of the tournament. It was not because he beat the other roosters, but because his inner strength brought peace and harmony to all who were near.

Four Horses

There is a zen saying that there are four types of horses. The first type of horse will run when you ask it to run. The second type of horse will run when you show it the whip. The third type of horse will run when you crack the whip in the air, and the fourth type of horse will run only when you beat it with the whip.

People are the same way. Some people will do exactly what you ask them to do when you ask them to do it. Other people will need to be told that there are consequences then they will do what you ask them to do. Yet other people will have to be threatened with the consequences. And, for the last group of people the consequences will have to be imposed and then they will do what you ask them to do.

You will encounter every one of these people in your life, and how you handle them determines where you fall in the lineup. It is important to understand the difference between these four types of people and how your everyday interactions will pan out. Pay careful attention to everyone around you and note who to watch.

Our Guiding Principles

Gichin Funakoshi's Five Rules

1. **You must be deadly serious in training.** Pay attention to what you are learning, because it might save your life someday. Don't fool around when Sensei is explaining a technique.

2. **Train with both heart and soul without worrying about theory.** Don't get too caught up in the details of what you are learning. It is more important that you take the lessons to heart and apply them in everyday life, than spending hours trying to get every single detail perfect.

3. **Avoid self-conceit and dogmatism.** Don't think too highly of your technique or hound other students to be more like you. You should concentrate on being humble about your abilities and helping others.

4. **Try to see yourself as you truly are and try to adopt what is meritous in others.** Don't have illusions about your skill. Accept your flaws, and work to see the best in others. Learn how to achieve the character goals you set and remember how much you still have to learn.

5. **Abide by the rules of ethics in your daily life, whether in public or private.** Be the same person in school or work as you are at home. Don't lie and cheat with your family members, and be perfectly honest at work and school. Be true to yourself and full of integrity.

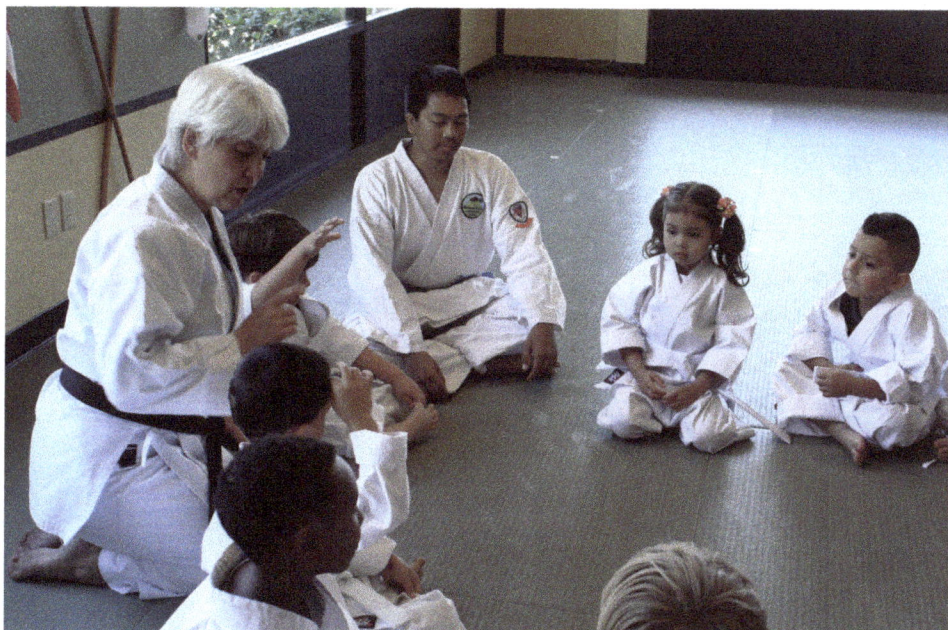

The Dojo Creed and How it Applies to Your Life

Seek Perfection of Character: This principle is not asking you to be perfect; it is a search for perfection. No one is perfect. Quite frankly, it is impossible to be perfect. It is possible to be very, very good at something. What's truly important, however, is that you consider what you do, what its long-term effect might be, and adjust your behavior when you realize that you're off the mark. This idea – that you can become a better person – is the foundation for all of our training.

Be Faithful: This principle means that you must believe in yourself. You must believe that you can succeed at what you're setting out to do. Without this belief in yourself, your success will not be in your hands, but in the hands of chance. Henry Ford, founder of the Ford Motor Company, said, "Whether a man thinks he can do something, or whether he thinks he can't do something, either way he's right." The way you think about something determines your ultimate success.

Observe the way you think about what you're about to do. If necessary, adjust your thinking before you start. If you can't, then reconsider whether or not you should do it. Then once you decide to do something: become an engineer, climb a mountain, get married, have kids, whatever it might be; continue to believe that you can do it despite trials and hardship. If you're only willing to try something, then you're setting yourself up to fail at it. As Yoda, the Jedi Master of Star Wars fame, said, "Do or do not. There is no try." But if you continue to believe in yourself and you're willing to give it everything you've got – your life if necessary – then you stand a far greater chance of succeeding.

Endeavor: This is the principle of persistence, of not easily letting go. You are willing to continue on even when faced with enormous obstacles, even when those who were with you at the start abandon you or turn against you. This principle challenges you to take on things that are bigger than yourself and continue until you succeed. When you do this, you will be transformed.

If you desire to be more than mediocre, accept the challenges that come your way. If you continually back down from challenges, you will be beaten down. You will start to feel weak and take on the mentality of a victim. We can assure you, this is not where you want to go.

Respect Others: Respect means to be seen and properly accepted. Consider this: You're walking down the street and a person walks right by you without saying hello, or giving any indication that you exist. Then a second person comes your way, looks at you and says hello. You say hello back, then you both walk on. How do you feel about each of these two people? You most likely feel neutral towards the first person and accepted by the second. Now which way is a better way to go through life? Ignoring people and having them feel nothing towards you, or respecting people and having them feel good about you? You decide; then act accordingly.

Refrain from Violent Behavior: This is about controlling your mind, body, and spirit. Remember that conflict begins in the mind with negative thoughts you may have about others or yourself. Thinking that you want harm to come to yourself or someone else is a form of violence even if you don't act on it. If you engage regularly in this way of thinking, you are setting yourself up for trouble.

We live in a country where people value freedom. Even so, people who think differently than you, and feel that you are harming them, can take your freedoms away. These people will restrict your freedom. The less you control yourself, the more successful they will be. In order to prevent others from confining your freedom, gain control over your mind, body and spirit. To put it another way: Either you can control yourself… Or others will control you.

Niju Kun

The Niju Kun are the twenty precepts of Gichin Funakoshi, the father of modern day karate. They are a more in depth study of the principles contained in the Dojo Creed and the Five Rules.

1. **Do not forget that karate starts and finishes with a bow:** Respect means to see and properly accept someone. Bowing is a way to show someone that they are seen and properly accepted.

    In order to respect others, you need to respect yourself first. A person who does not respect him or herself will come across as insincere when they attempt to show respect to someone else.

    What if you respect yourself but the other person is not, in your opinion, worthy of respect?

    We share the same emotions with other human beings. We all feel good when someone shows respect to us. When you respect another person, even if they are not worthy of your respect, you make them feel good. You are opening the door for that person to respect him or herself, and become a person who is worthy of your respect.

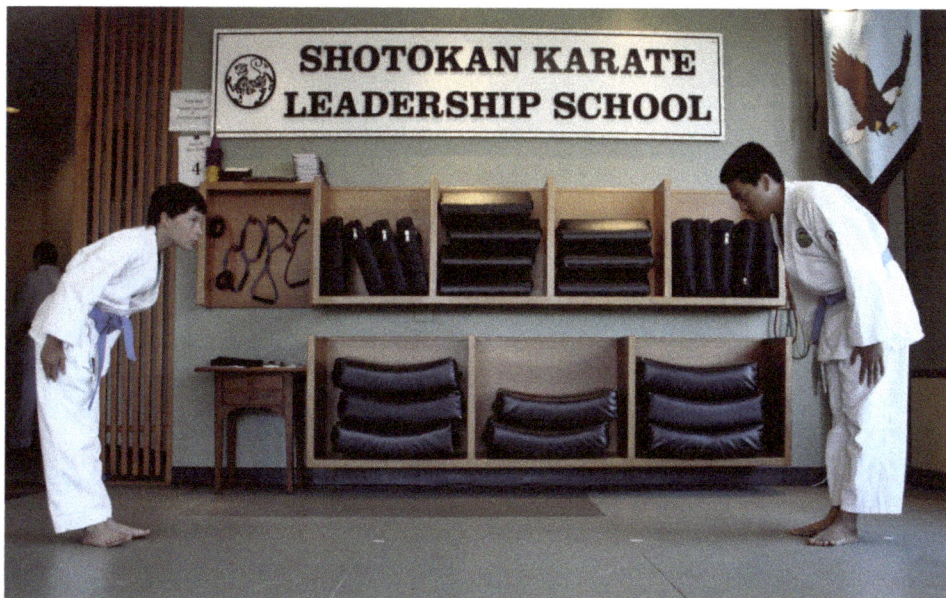

2. **In karate, never attack first:** This principle addresses the fact that you must never attack first with your mind. This means that you should not think about hurting anyone in any way. At the same time, another person might decide to attack you. If this happens, then you can make the first move to stop them. You would be physically attacking first, but you did not mentally attack first, because you never thought about or decided to harm the other person.

   If someone is angry with you and there's a stick nearby, and they look angrily at you, then at the stick. They look back at you, then reach for the stick. It's obvious that they're about to club you with the stick. You would be foolish if you waited for them to hit you before you attacked them. You should act first to prevent them from attacking you.

   Patience, tolerance and self control are demonstrations of strength. Tolerate what you see as weaknesses and inconsistencies in others. Be patient with yourself and others and control your actions and reactions. These are signs of true strength.

   Weak individuals strike first with little provocation. The strong restrain themselves as long as possible. We practice this in class during sparring, when we learn to wait as long as possible before responding to an attack.

3. **One who practices karate must follow the way of justice:** Justice is doing what is right in the right way. Following the way of justice means living your life considering what the right thing to do is, then doing it the right way.

   A good place to start is your own moral compass when you find yourself in a quandary. Ask yourself what the right thing to do is, then listen for the answer. You will learn to follow the way of justice as you practice, if you strive to perform your technique as close as possible to the ideal. You will be doing what is right in the right way. Every time you practice this you will develop a clearer understanding of what is right and what is wrong.

4. **First, you must know yourself. Only then can you know others:** Knowing yourself in mind, body and spirit will give you insight into other people. Without self-knowledge, your basis for understanding others is incomplete. Be aware of the state of your mind. Are you worried and filled with doubt, or are you experiencing peace and serenity? Know your body. Are you sick or healthy, weak or strong, in pain or comfortable?

   Know your spirit. How are you coping with life's challenges? Are you being overcome by the sheer enormity of life or are you taking life on and meeting it on your own terms?

   Of these three, your spirit, or life force, is the most important. It is what makes you alive. Knowing the condition of your spirit at all times is critically important to your success. Deep breathing, relaxation exercises, and focused effort will do wonders to bring your spirit back up.

   To paraphrase *The Art of War* by Sun Tsu: If you know yourself and your opponent, you need not fear any battle. If you only know yourself, and not your opponent, you have a 50/50 chance of victory. If you don't know yourself or your opponent you are in grave danger.

5. **Spirit and mind are more important than technique:** Your point of view and the way your brain processes information are true indicators of what you

will do in life. If you think it's important to treat other people respectfully, then you will behave accordingly.

Your mind and your spirit determine what you can and will do with your technique. It is important that you ask yourself what the best way to develop your mind and spirit is, then carry it out.

Your mind can be trained effectively by considering a problem that exists in the world and creating a solution. A simple solution will do for a simple problem, but a more complex solution will be needed for a more complex problem.

To create a solution for a complex problem, determine what the outcome will look like, arrange the core elements, build the structure, and put the final touches on. While working on it, think of it as a puzzle and you have to figure out which way the pieces fit together. When you retrieve the solution, the accomplishment will be that much sweeter.

Don't let others think for you. If someone expresses their opinion about something, think about what they said, and if it doesn't make sense, question it. If it stands up to scrutiny, then it's probably sound, but if it doesn't, don't adopt that point of view. It's most likely faulty.

6. **You must be ready to release your mind:** Be in a constant state of readiness to let go of what you have. A way to understand this is to examine the process an archer goes through to shoot his or her bow.

After an archer has drawn back and taken aim, all that's left for him to do is release and the arrow flies on its way to the target. For this to work effectively, the archer must be in a balanced state between tension and relaxation. Too relaxed, and the arrow won't reach it's target, too much tension, and the bow could break, the shot could be erratic, or the archer might shoot himself. Ideally, the archer would be in a state that has enough tension to drive the arrow to the target and enough relaxation to maintain control.

Imagine an individual whose body and mind are relaxed– he or she would be lethargic and unable to function. Now imagine an individual whose body and mind are tensed – they would be a maniac, full of energy and out of control. Neither one of these states are in balance, let alone high functioning.

Peak performance requires all aspects of your being– mind, body, and spirit– to be in balance, running smoothly in every aspect. To achieve this state, you must be ready to react, and ready to let go of all your emotions and limitations.

7. **Misfortune comes out of idleness:** Why do some people mess up when they have so much going for them? This principle explains that this happens when a person idles away their time, instead of developing their capabilities.

If messing up is the result of idleness, then the opposite must also be true. Exerting an effort to better yourself, or applying your energy towards a worthy cause will bring good fortune. If you want a good life and to feel fulfilled, take an interest in the world around you and when you see something needs fixing help make it right.

8. **Don't think that what you learn in karate can't be used outside the dojo:** You will feel empowered by taking karate. You will learn the freedom to say yes or no to opportunities and challenges. Your whole life will change, and

you will become a different person– more confident and sure of yourself. Every technique you earn has an application in real life. Karate will help you learn to see things in new ways. Don't confine your ways of thinking in boxes. You can apply what you learn in life outside of karate to karate and what you learn in karate to life outside the dojo.

9. **It will take all your life to learn karate:** A lesson learned today is forgotten tomorrow, unless you relearn it tomorrow. It is human nature to forget. If you attend a lecture, you will remember only about 10% of what you heard. You have to experience things many times before you won't forget them.

   The potential lessons you can learn from karate are infinite. You could practice every day for the rest of your life and still not learn everything there is to learn. Practice until every cell in your body absorbs the lesson you are working on, even if you feel like you've done it the best you could already. There is always room for improvement.

10. **Put karate into your everyday living. That is how to see its true beauty:** Consider three things: everyday living, beauty, and karate. Everyday living is everything that is not karate. Beauty is something that is attractive. It could be anything you experience, or an idea that is just perfect.

    When you apply karate to your everyday life, it's not about the moves you learn, but the qualities gained from practicing karate such as courage, courtesy, integrity, humility and self-control. These are the things that will bring beauty to karate and your life.

11. **Karate is like hot water; if you do not give it continuous heat, it will become cold:** Water is an amazing element. It flows, stands still, destroys, and heals. Without water, we would be dead in a matter of days.

    When it is hot, it can cook our food and warm our hands, but if it escapes from its container, it can burn and cause extensive damage. If the heat is taken away, it will cool, just like many other elements.

    Karate is the same. Like water, it can adapt to circumstances. When it is used properly, it can help, and if it is used improperly, it can destroy. Without continuous practice, your karate skills will dull and grow stale.

12. **Do not cling to the idea of winning; it is the idea of not losing that is necessary:** The most common view of success requires you to win at everything: Your passion, your hobby, your work, and your everyday life.

    But martial arts teaches that if you cling to the idea of winning, you are holding on to something that is incomplete. Monkeys are captured sometimes by placing meat in a heavy jar with a small opening in it. This opening will only allow their open hand to pass through, not their closed fist. A monkey will reach in, grab the meat, and not be able to get his hand out. When the monkey's captor approaches, they refuse to let go of the meat so they can escape. Greed is their downfall.

    Holding tightly to the idea of winning will cause you to miss out on something greater: Your freedom. Focus on not losing instead of on winning, and you will have freedom and success.

    If you remove losing from the picture, all that remains is winning.

13. **Move according to your opponent:** When working with other people, start by understanding them and why they do what they do. When the time is right, you can create and suggest solutions to problems. It's not that you can't create change, but how you go about doing it is important if you want to succeed. In battle, become one with your opponent, keeping up with them until time and circumstances are favorable to making a change. Be aware of what those around you are doing so you can know the right time to do or say something.

14. **In conflict, you must discern the vulnerable from the invulnerable points:** You have strong points and weak points. Sometimes your strong points appear to be your weak points and your weak points appear to be your strong points. It is important to know the difference yourself, even if others can't.

    When you are certain of your strengths and weaknesses, you will recognize others' strengths and weaknesses. If you don't know your strengths and weaknesses, or if you fool yourself into believing your weaknesses are your strengths, you will not see them clearly in others.

15. **Consider your opponent's legs and arms as you would lethal swords:** John D. Rockefeller III, one of the wealthiest men in America in his time, died in a car accident caused by a joyriding 14 year-old. Anyone and anything can be a lethal opponent, even a child. There are people who have died from a paper cut getting infected. Any time you find yourself in a conflict, the result could be fatal for either one of you. Act accordingly.

16. **Be aware at all times that you have millions of potential opponents:** You need to be constantly aware, but not paranoid. If you repeatedly told a young child that there were bad people outside waiting for them, you would instill fear in that child. There are bad people in the world, but there is also an overwhelming amount of good people. It is better to tell the truth and have them be aware of bad people, than tilt the scales and have a fear-filled child afraid of their own shadow.

    You are developing the skills to deal with potential opponents, then going out into the world to do what you need to do, facing those opponents without fear when you encounter them.

    The reverse of this is true as well. If there are millions of potential opponents, then there are also millions of opportunities to move ahead and gain new friends.

17. **Postured stance is for beginners; later comes naturalness:** When you begin a new endeavor, you learn and develop new ways of doing a certain thing. After doing it for a while, it begins to feel natural. When you go to a new school or start a new job, it can be awkward and weird as you adjust to a new place. However, as time goes by, you will become more comfortable with your surroundings, even enjoy them.

    Learning correct form can be difficult and even painful. Practice with the knowledge that it will get easier and more natural to your body as you continue.

18. **Kata is about correct and proper form; engaging in a real fight is something else:** Correct form came from thousands of years of determining

the most effective way to deliver a technique to a target with maximum speed and power. A martial artist will spend many years refining their skills, so they can move effectively in the blink of an eye. Their goal is to reach a high level of control over their body.

In a real fight, movement must be spontaneous. Proper form is the basis for spontaneous movement, but the movement itself must be done without thinking about how perfect it looks. If your form is properly developed, it will support quick, powerful movements. If your form is weak, it won't.

Practice correct form during training, but in actual combat, let go of the restraints of correct form and move freely. Your preservation is more important than a perfect forward stance when it's life and death.

19. **Do not forget a) strength and weakness of power; b) contraction and expansion of body, and c) rhythm of techniques:** It's easy to think that power is only being strong, but to fully understand power you must know when power should be used lightly or heavily. Sometimes, a show of power is needed, but other times, it only takes a small amount to achieve your task.

Your muscles do two things, contracting and expanding. Both of these movements can be used to increase the effectiveness of your techniques. In life, opportunities appear and disappear. Everything flourishes and dies in its own time. If you understand this, then you will understand when change is coming and be prepared for anything.

Rhythm is movement that follows a prescribed beat or tempo. Each technique has its own time frame. Some techniques can be executed in one tenth of a second. Others will take five seconds. Once you understand the time it will take to complete a technique, then you can give it exactly the time it needs before moving to the next one.

The things you do take time to complete, just as the sun rising and setting happens over the course of a day. If you want to succeed, you need to learn to be patient. Understand the timing and rhythm of life and you will achieve great things.

20. **Always create and devise:** Imagination is your greatest tool. You have an infinite supply of it, and you should make a habit of using it every day. The world is a better place when good people like you use their imaginations to create solutions to problems mankind faces.

Keep this knowledge in your focus, and you will be renewed daily.

The Twelve Traits of a Shoka Leader

We want to help you become a great leader through the training we give you. We want you to become the best version of yourself, and by concentrating on these character traits as you move through the ranks will allow you to become courageous, courteous, honest, humble, and exercise self-control. You will also learn to be trustworthy, endeavoring, responsible, cooperative, just, compassionate, and creative. Every week, you will have an assignment to utilize the character trait of the month in some way.
The purpose of each trait is laid out below:

Courage Instill the importance of being strong in the face of danger.

Courtesy The importance of respecting yourself and others.

Integrity Instill honesty and the need to think, speak, and act as one.

Humility Recognize that you are small in comparison to the vast universe.

Self-Control Understand the need to control your mind, body and spirit.

Trust Understand the meaning of trust, placing confidence in someone or something, and the need to be trustworthy.

Endeavor Begin to develop the inner strength necessary to continue on despite facing great obstacles.

Responsibility Begin to develop the ability to respond to circumstances and fulfill your duties to others.

Cooperation Understand the importance of teams and how to work well with others.

Justice Learn to perceive the difference between right and wrong and develop the strength necessary to stand on the side of justice despite the consequences.

Compassion Open up to the pain others may be feeling and work to alleviate that pain.

Creativity Understand that your greatest strength lies in your ability to imagine a better world, and begin to create that new world.

Manners

Rules and procedures help control what happens on the training floor, and manners have to do with what happens off the training floor. There are generally accepted manners: Respecting others, listening to what they have to say, not interrupting, etc. Good manners are your first line of self-defense. You should always be considerate of others and willing to hear them out. If you are kind to others and don't antagonize your peers, you can prevent situations from becoming volatile. Even if someone is threatening you, you can often talk your way out of it.

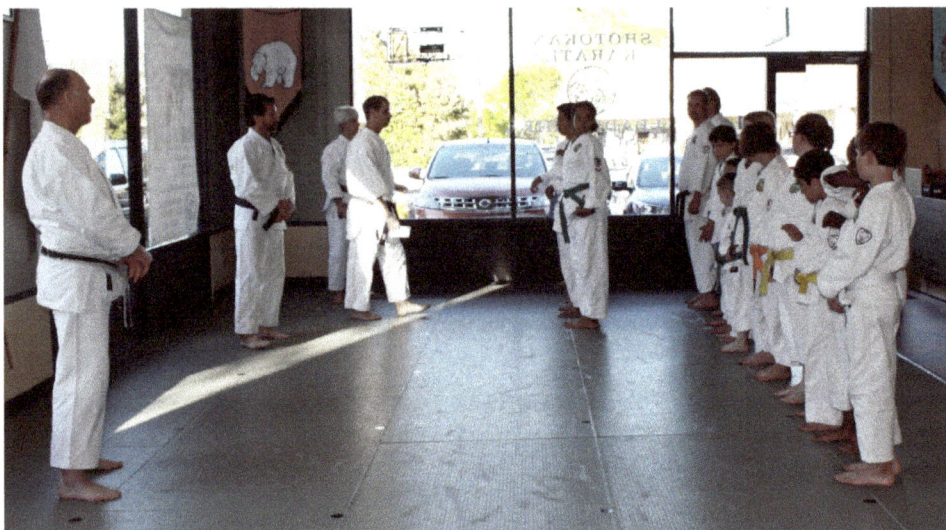

Besides the manners that can help you outside the school, there are also manners more specific to Shotokan Karate Leadership School®. They include the following:

7 Points of respect: Yes, Sir. Yes, Ma'am. No, Sir. No, Ma'am. Please. Thank you. Excuse me.

Remove your shoes and socks before going on the mat. Put them side-by-side, against the wall. If there is already a line of shoes against the wall, you can put your shoes underneath a bench or in another line against the previous line of shoes. Store your other stuff out of the way. This includes jackets, hats, and bags. Put them in your school gear bag, then set it out of the way or in the back.

Bow before entering and leaving the room. The standing bow starts with your heels together and your toes at a 30-degree angle, your back straight and head up. Your eyes are looking straight ahead, shoulders relaxed, and hands held open along the side of the legs You should have the sensation that you are breathing from the lower abdomen. From this position, bend your body forward from your hips, keeping your back straight. Bring your eyes down to about 8 feet in front of you. If you are bowing to a person, drop your eyes from their face to their lower body. Upon completion of the bow, return to the upright position. The bow should take about 3 seconds total.

Be on time for class. If you're catching a ride with someone else, make sure they know you're expected to be on time. Give them a schedule if they need one. If you can't be on time for class, follow the late procedures – put your attendance card on the instructor table, sit in seiza and have your own period of meditation, bow when you're finished, then, if the warm up exercises are still going on, get up and join the class. If the instructor has begun to teach, then, wait until you get permission to join the class.

Introduce yourself to others and greet visitors. Look them in the eye, say hello, and put your hand out. Tell them your name, ask them theirs, shake their hand when they offer it, and tell them it's nice to meet them. Do this with a smile on your face and a cheerful attitude.

Note: If they don't offer their hand, just lower yours and continue introducing yourself. Sometimes a person doesn't want to shake hands because of a belief they have, or they don't like germs. Don't insist and don't take it as a sign of disrespect.

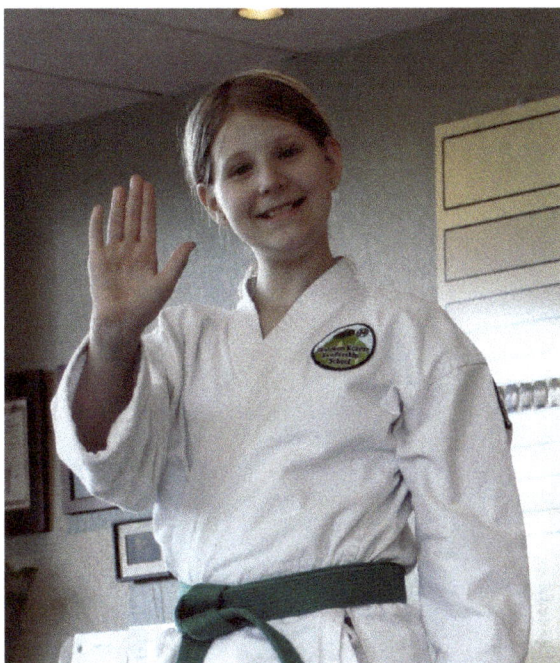

Rules and Procedures

Rules and procedures let you know what to do when you're on the training floor. Procedures are general, where rules are specific. It is important that you understand the intent of the rules. They exist to ensure the environment on the training floor supports the development of your mind, body, and spirit.

Rules

1. **Safety first.** Show spirit, enthusiasm, respect, and good sportsmanship at all times and do nothing that could endanger the well-being of your classmates.
2. **Do not chew gum or eat food on the mat.** Gum or food could cause you to bite your tongue or if it fell out of your mouth, it could mess up the floor. Please be respectful.
3. **Do not talk during class.** Talking is a distraction to others. If you have a question, raise your hand. If it's a good time, your instructor will call on you. If it isn't, he will ask you to put your hand down.
4. **Do not excuse yourself from class without the instructor's permission.** If you must leave early, get permission BEFORE class starts. If you have to leave suddenly due to an emergency, please attempt to leave without disturbing the class. Notify your instructor about the emergency and leave quickly and quietly.
5. **Wear a clean, white, SKLS karate-gi**. Keep your uniform clean, wrinkle-free, and in good repair.
6. **Keep your fingernails and toenails short; do not wear watches or jewelry while training**. There is some contact made in class and long nails or hard objects could hurt another student.
7. **Respond quickly to instructions.** Never argue with your instructor. If you don't understand, ask a question, and your instructor will answer it. If his or her answer doesn't satisfy you, ask another question. If he has the time, he or she will engage in a conversation with you to help you understand, or arrange another time to speak with you. All of our instructors want you to understand what they are teaching.

Procedures

1. **Attendance card:** If it's your first class of the week, it will be in the A box. If it's your second or third class, it will be in the B box. If you haven't attended for a week or more, it will be in the C box. The cards will be collected after everyone has lined up.
2. **When you are late for class** if you are not in line to sit down when the last person sits after the command 'seiza' is given. Sit down at the back of the room, have your own period of meditation, bow, and if the warm up period is still going on, join the class. If the warm up period is over and the instructor has begun to teach, wait for a signal from the instructor to enter the class, then join quickly and quietly with as little interruption to the other students as possible.
3. **Notify your instructor when you will be absent** due to illness, injury, or vacation.

Class Commands

Line up: When the command to line up is given, do so quickly and quietly in order of rank. Do not line up until every rank above you has lined up. Often, students will walk in the door shortly before line up and there will not be enough space for them to get in line. Student leaders will line up in front of the students and the instructors will line up in front of the student leaders.

Otagi ni rei: When the command to turn around and face our guests is given, do so promptly. At the command, *otagi ni rei*, bow to the guests, then turn around again. This is done to show respect to your parents and grandparents.

Seiza: When the command to sit in 'seiza' (pronounced say-za), the sitting/kneeling position, is given, the highest-ranking student sits down first, then the rest of the students sit down in order of rank. If you are right-handed, put your right knee on the floor first, and if you are left-handed, put your left knee down first. Put your other knee down, so you are kneeling, but the rest of your body is upright. Cross your right foot over your left foot if you are right-handed, and the opposite if you are left-handed. Sit down, keeping your back straight. Keep your arms by your sides until you are seated and then move your hands to your thighs and turn them inward at a 30-degree angle. Straighten your back and look down at the floor about 3 feet in front of you.

Mokuso: When the command to meditate is given – 'mokuso' (pronounced mock-so) – close your eyes halfway and take a deep breath in through your nose. Let the sensation circle around in your head, push the sensation down to your lower abdomen, and hold it there. Slowly breathe out through your mouth until about 80% of the air has left your body, then start the process again with another breath in. Clear your mind completely and concentrate only on your breathing.

Mokuso yame: When the command to stop meditating is given (mokuso yame), open your eyes fully. This is when the dojo creed will be recited at the end of class.

Shomen ni rei: When the command to bow to the front is given (shomen ni rei), place both of your hands simultaneously flat on the floor in front of you at about a 30 degree angle inward, look down between your hands, lower your body until your head is about a foot off the floor, then return to seiza. Altogether this should take about 3 seconds.

The reason Gichin Funakoshi and Masatoshi Nakayama's pictures are on the front wall is because they made major contributions to the art of Shotokan Karate. They were the founders of karate as we know it, and showing respect to them is like showing respect to your parents and grandparents who have done so much to make life better for you. The American and the Japanese Flags are also on the front wall, because this is the United States, but Shotokan Karate came from Japan. Shotokan Karate Leadership School® believes it is our duty to do all we can to maintain good relations between the U.S. and Japan.

Sensei ni rei: When the command to bow to the instructor is given (sensei ni rei), repeat the same procedure. This is to show respect to your teacher, who will help you learn everything you can.

Your Uniform

Your uniform or gi (pronounced gee) is an important part of being a karate student. After you have practiced in class a few times and felt the excitement of training, you will reach a point where just putting your gi on will make you feel ready for action. After you earn your first belt, putting your belt on will enhance that feeling.

Your uniform should be worn with pride, so take good care of it. Wash it regularly, and hang it up or iron it so it remains wrinkle free. Have your sleeves and cuffs hemmed or fold them under tightly so they are 2 to 3 inches above your wrists and ankles. Your uniform represents your respect for yourself, your instructor, your fellow students, and your school. It should be treated as such. When you wear your uniform, wear the whole uniform – pants, top and belt – and make sure that everything is properly tied. If you are only half-dressed, you are only half-prepared. This is true when you wear your uniform in public as well.

When dressing put your pants on first and if they have a drawstring, make sure the loops are in the front. If it has an elastic waistband, there should be a pull string at the front. Tuck your strings into your waistband. Put the top on next. It has two flaps and is worn much like a jacket. Each flap has two strings. The middle string is near the side of your body and the end string is at the end of the flap. Fold the right flap across your body and tie the right end string to the left middle string with a bowknot. You'll want to get out of your uniform when you've finished training and a bowknot will let you do that easily. Fold the left flap across your body and tie the left end string to the right middle string.

Now it's time to put on your belt. Find the middle of your belt by holding it up in front of you, then put the middle of the belt just below your bellybutton and wrap it around behind you and back in front. You now have one end of the belt in each hand. Take the end of the belt in your left hand and fold it across the middle of the belt, and then take the end of the belt in your right hand and fold it on top of that. Loop it under both strands of the belt. This end of the belt is now in your left hand and is coming out from under the two strands of the belt diagonally, while the other end of the belt in your right hand is coming down diagonally. Fold the right end across the middle of the belt and make a loop, then take the left end and fold it over the top of the loop. Weave it up and through the loop. Voila! You now have a properly tied belt that a black belt would be proud of!

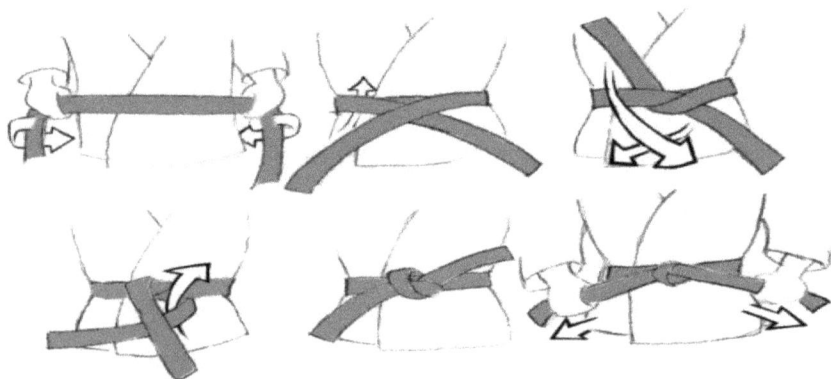

Community Service

Why You Need to Learn to Lead

To make the world a better place. The world needs more people to step up and lead, especially in this age of technology. Everyone is glued to their phones or video games, too concerned with getting likes on their selfie or reaching the next level. The world would be a better place if everyone paid attention to old ladies struggling with their groceries and lost children. You can be a leader, humble and aware of those in need. It is vitally important for you to care about those around you enough to lead them to a better way of life. If you don't step up, who will?

Your community service work begins at the dojo. You will be asked to help clean, talk to parents, introduce yourself to others, help younger students, assist us in promoting the school, and do things to help around the office and the school.

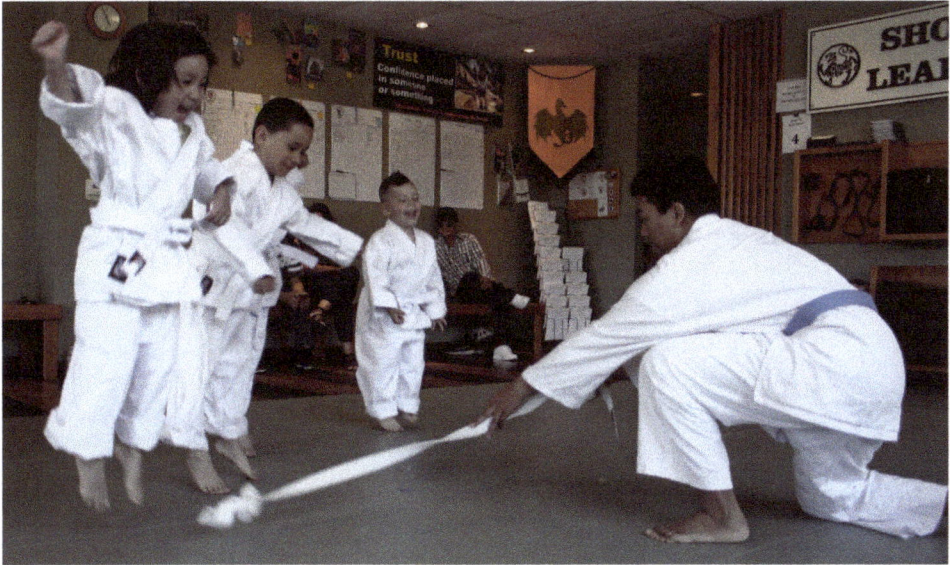

The Shoka Way of Leadership

Why Shotokan Karate Leadership School® is an Ideal Way to Learn to Lead:

At SKLS, you learn practical life lessons and how to live a successful life filled with compassion and integrity. Every time you come to class, you will learn more about becoming a strong leader who can change the world. There are years of experience both in life and karate under our instructor's belts. We use a time honored, scientifically supported, systematic approach to help you achieve your goals.

Setting Goals

Step One: Visualizing the Goal

In order to set a goal, you have to know what you want. It's not important in the first stages to know how you're going to get there. All you need to do in the beginning is imagine yourself achieving that goal. If your goal is to run a 5k, visualize the run and crossing the finish line. If your goal is getting your black belt, then imagine being handed your black belt and putting it on. If you can see yourself doing it, you can do it.

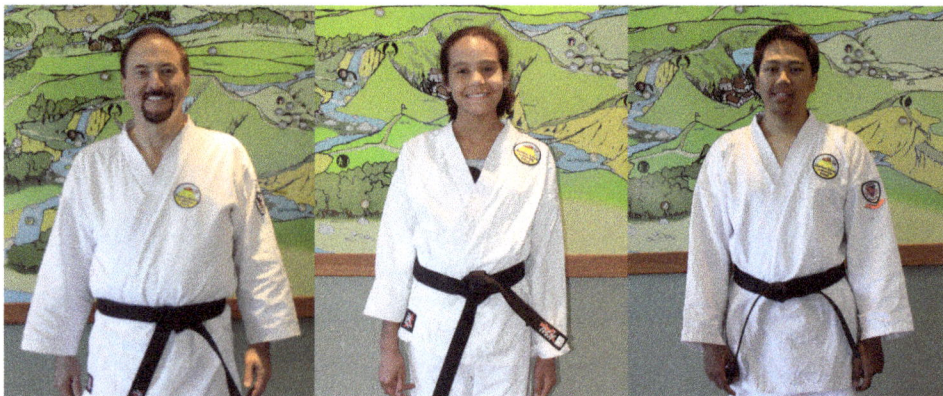

Step Two: Self-Talk About the Goal

You will not achieve what you set out to do if you cannot believe in yourself. Telling yourself every day that you are horrible at taking tests will not help your test-taking ability. Instead, look yourself in the mirror every day and say, "I am great at taking tests. I am not nervous. I can do this." Positive self-talk is the best way to not only help yourself achieve your goal, but also to have better self-esteem and a happier life. For more information read What to Say When You Talk to Yourself, by Shad Helmstetter.

Step Three: Support in Reaching Your Goal

In order to accomplish what you are working towards, you need the support of those around you. Your teacher at school helps you get your homework done, your friends help you when you need someone to talk to, and your sensei helps you reach your black belt. Everyone around you is likely willing to help you earn an achievement. Ask for help, even if it's just having someone tell you that your goal is a good thing to work towards. The people in your life care about you and want you to succeed. The very best way to get the support you need is to give it first. Start by asking the important people in your life what you can do to help them, this will pave the way for them to help you.

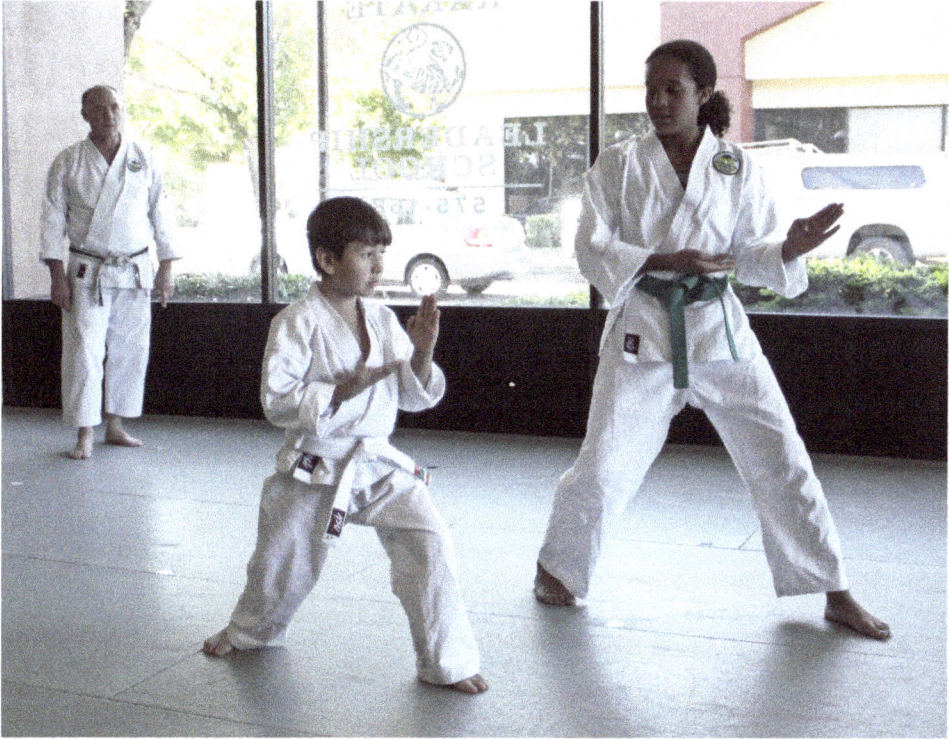

Step Four: Commitment

In order to complete your goal, you have to be committed to it. The Oxford English Dictionary defines commitment as "the state or quality of being dedicated to a cause or activity; a pledge or undertaking." In other terms, commitment is a promise you make, usually to yourself. If your commitment is weak, you will give up at the first sign of trouble. But if your commitment is strong, you will keep going no matter how hard it gets. Making a commitment is extremely important. It can cause you to learn things you wouldn't have without the promise you made to yourself. The person who will be most disappointed about you not reaching your goal will be yourself.

The Four Levels

The Black Belt Shoka Leader Program is built on two beliefs. First, that there is an extraordinary leader within every person, and proper teaching, support, and training will awaken the leader in you, enabling you to transform the world. Second, that the secret to extraordinary leadership can be found in the art of karate and will reveal itself to those who persist in looking for it.

How the transformation from ordinary person to extraordinary leader happens can be understood by examining what happens in the Black Belt Shoka Leader Program.

Level 1: Green – Independently Motivated Self-Starter

In the first year of this program, you will learn to fulfill your responsibilities without being told. You will learn to set goals, create plans, and follow through and attain those goals. You will do this because you want to, and are independently motivated to be successful. You will become an excellent student.

Level 2: Purple – Productive Team Member

In the second year, you will learn to work with all kinds of people, create synergy, and be responsible for your own results. This is an important quality that many employers look for.

Level 3: Brown – Result-Oriented Team Leader

In the third year, you will learn to assemble a team, identify strengths and weakness in that team, make appropriate assignments, and create the results that the team must achieve.

Level 4: Black – Humble Servant Leader of People

In year four, you will learn to work with several teams and take responsibility for creating the results that all the teams need to gain. You will also learn to work with large, diverse group of individuals, assemble them into teams, and achieve the results the school needs. This level includes public speaking, presentation skills, stage presence, and advanced teaching skills.

Our Promise

Upon completion of our program we will awaken the extraordinary leader in you – the leader who can dream, think, tell your story, and lead.

Teamwork

Being a Productive Team Member

The most important thing to do as a team member is to listen to your leader. Follow the directions they give you to the best of your abilities, but don't be afraid to ask for help. Do not skip out on your responsibilities, or you will not receive respect from your leader and fellow teammates. If you consistently fulfill your responsibilities and work well with your teammates, you will be rewarded and may even become a leader of your own team.

Being a Result-Oriented Team Leader

Two of the most important things to know as a team leader are the strengths and weaknesses of every member of your team. Be aware of any physical or mental disabilities that team members have, and work with them as best you can. Do not take advantage of your position as a leader. Leaders are humble and think about the good of their team above their own selfish desires. You will have to make both easy and difficult decisions as a team leader, and you need to be prepared to handle both.

Student Leaders

Leadership is the ability to affect change in yourself and the world around you. Leading requires a clear mind, a compelling vision, an above average ability to communicate the vision to others, an uncanny ability to read others, the ability to admit mistakes, the patience of a saint and a fierce determination to do whatever it takes, for as long as it takes. However, leadership also takes practice and failure.

If you are eager to discover how to get started in leadership, there are plenty of positions available here in our school. From planning activities to becoming an instructor, program director, school director, school owner, or leader in our young and growing organization. You can learn and teach valuable life skills surrounded by your peers in a safe and familiar environment.

Class Leader

The Class Leader is qualified to assist in beginning and intermediate classes. Being a Class Leader leads to a greater feelings of confidence and improves the student's technical skills. Teaching leads to feelings of satisfaction by helping others. The minimum age and rank is 8 years old and 6th kyu Green Belt.

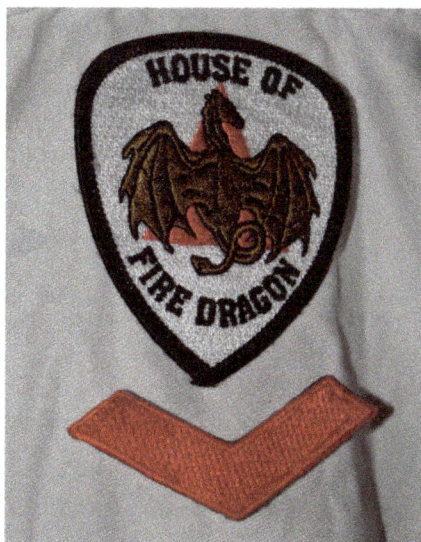

The Class Leader reports directly to the Instructor and is a member of the Student Leaders Council. A red chevron will be added to the left shoulder below the House Patch. The Class Leaders line up in a row in front of the regular students and to the right.

House Leader

A House Leader organizes and conducts fun house activities. Ice skating, roller skating, birthday parties, movie nights, pizza parties, events in the park or a trip to the beach are imagined, planned, and carried out by the House Leader. House Leaders must be at least 11 years old and hold a minimum rank of 5th kyu Blue Belt. House Leaders have the responsibility of making the final decision about how the house points are spent. Each house will also have an adult House Leader who will be available to assist the student House Leader when needed.

A House Leader wears a brown bar on their right shoulder about 2 inches below the shoulder seam, lines up in a row in front of and to the left of the students, and they are a member of the Student Leaders Council.

School Leader

The School Leader assists with school operations and the vitally important function of attracting new students. This could be a starting place for future income and a wonderful start to an impressive resumé. The minimum age and rank for this role is 11 years old and a 4th kyu purple belt.

This position reports to and is directed by the Program Director. The School Leader is in a rotating position of Chair of the Student Leaders Council. He or she wears a black bar on their right shoulder 1 inch below the shoulder seam. The School Leader lines up in a row in front of the regular students in the center of the room.

Student Instructors

Assistant Instructor

An Assistant Instructor is qualified to teach beginning and intermediate students. The minimum age and rank is 9 years old and a 3rd kyu Brown Belt. Assistant Instructors report directly to the Instructor. The Assistant Instructor lines up in front of the student leaders and slightly back and to the right of the Junior Instructor. Assistant Instructors are members of the School Board of Review and wear two red chevrons on the left shoulder below the House Patch.

Junior Instructor

A Junior Instructor is qualified to teach all levels and programs of youth below age 15. The minimum age is 10, and the minimum rank is 1st dan Black Belt. This position reports directly to the Instructor.

The Junior Instructor is a member of the School Board of Review and the Instructional Board. Junior Instructors are no longer members of a house, but instead belong to the instructor corps, and as such, wear two red chevrons below the Instructor Patch. Junior Instructors stand slightly back and to the right of the Instructor.

Instructor

An Instructor is qualified to teach all levels and all programs. The minimum age is 16, and the minimum rank is 1st dan Black Belt. This position reports directly to the Head Instructor.

The Instructor is a member of the School Board of Review and the Instructional Board. Instructors are no longer members of a house, but instead belong to the instructor corps, and as such, wear two red chevrons below the Instructor Patch. Instructors stand slightly back and to the right of the Senior Instructor.

How We Train Leaders

Commands

Commands are to be followed as quickly as possible. In order to become a leader, you must first become a good follower. Responding quickly is also essential in life-or-death situations. The development of quick reflexes can mean the difference between life and death. Training here is meant to help you in all aspects of your life, and you need to treat it as such.

Counting

As a student you learn to wait for the instructor or student leader to count before moving, and you learn to pay attention to the way they use their voice. As a leader you will learn how to count clearly and at the right time. Whether counting in Japanese or English, always use a powerful voice. You are directing others, and you should act like it.

Use of Voice

If you use a powerful voice, you are more likely to believe you are powerful. It tells other people to listen to you, that you have something important to say. A shrill or quiet voice informs others that you don't believe what you say or that you don't have confidence in what you are saying or doing. Pay attention to your tone of voice when directing others or asking questions. Your voice can be extremely transparent, and you should be careful what emotions you are expressing without realizing it.

Body Posture

Stand straight and tall at all times. Slouching and hunching your shoulders sends a message of defeat and laziness. Be in command of your surroundings and aware of your interactions with people. Poor posture tells others you don't care about yourself. Be proud of who you are and what you stand for.

The School

Here at Shotokan Karate Leadership School®, we are dedicated to improving the lives of our students, their families, and our community. Our instructors are experts in human development. We want you to feel respected and safe. Our goal is to push you to do your best, whether that means helping you learn the best way to practice or letting you know that you can do better. Please do not hesitate to voice any issues you might have. We will do our best to mediate the situation or explain why we do things a certain way.

Community Leadership

It's just as important to be a leader in Shotokan Karate Leadership School® as it is to be one outside of it. Find a way to get involved with a project to better your community. Go to your city's parks and recreation building and find out how you can help. Maybe you can plan some trees or clean up trash. Start a recycling drive or mow your neighbor's lawn for free. Be helpful in any way you can. Ask your teacher to give you projects to help in the classroom. The possibilities are endless once you set your mind to it.

Shotokan Karate

Warm up Exercises

You are expected to follow the warm up exercises as well as you can when you first start. Eventually, you will learn to lead them as a Class Leader. The warm up exercises help your muscles stretch and loosen so you won't pull anything when you participate in class.

Exercise	Command
Open your legs to the side and stretch down to the middle.	Open your legs. Down to the center.
Reach your left hand to your right foot and then your right hand to your left foot	Reach to your right foot. Reach to your left foot.
Straighten up and lean back.	Lean back.
Reach your left arm over the top of your head to the right side then reverse.	Over to your right side Over to your left side
Deeply bend your right leg while stretching the inside of your left leg. Do both sides.	Stretch the inside of your leg (right side) Reverse.
Deeply bend your left leg while stretching the back of your right leg. Do both sides.	Back side. Reverse.
Deeply bend your right leg while coming up on the toes of your extended leg. Do both sides.	Up on your toes. Reverse.
Side splits with feet flat on the floor and toes pointed straight forward.	Side splits
Side splits. Lower your hips, arch back. Look back and over your right shoulder, then your left shoulder, and then straight back. Walk back on your heels and let your heels slide out.	Walk your hands out. Lower your hips. Arch back. Look back and over your right shoulder. Back and over your left shoulder. Straight back. Back on your heels. Let your heels slide out.
Front splits to the right and left sides.	Turn to your right side. Back to the center. Turn to the left side.
Back to side splits with the toes off the floor and slide the feet out.	Back to the center. Let your heels slide out.
Walk your hands back and sit down with your legs open wide.	Sit back.
Put your right hand on the floor with the palm up across in front of your body and reach over the top to your right foot. Do both sides.	Put your right hand across your lap and reach over to your right foot. Reverse.
Reach for your right foot with your right hand	Again to your right leg.

and grab your right ankle with your left hand and pull your chin towards your knee. Do both sides.	Grab your ankle and your foot. Chin to your knee. Reverse
Put your hands on the floor behind you and push yourself forward opening your legs as wide as they will go.	Push yourself forward.
Walk your fingers forward and lower your chest to the floor.	Walk your fingers out. Chest to the floor.
Bring your legs together and bounce your knees. Then point your toes, grab your ankles and pull yourself forward.	Bring your legs together. Bounce your knees. Point your toes. Grab your ankles pull yourself forward.
Flex your ankles back and reach for your toes.	Toes and ankles back. Reach for your toes.
Bring your feet in close with the sole of the feet together close to your body. Grab your ankles and use your elbows to push your knees to the floor. (Butterfly position)	Feet in close. Use your elbows push your knees down. Grab your toes, pull yourself forward.
Put your left leg in front while bending your right leg across your lap, grab your ankle and foot and pull your chin to your knee. Twist towards the back in the direction of bent right leg. Repeat on the other side.	Left leg in front. Grab your ankle and your foot. Chin to your knee. Twist to the back. Reverse. Chin to your knee. Twist to the back.
Reach forward bend your knees and turn them out to the sides with your feet turned in (frog stretch). Push your hips straight back. Turn to your right knee; then towards your left knee. Then straight back.	Stretch your hips. Push back. Over to your right knee. To your left knee. And again straight back.
Put your fists on the floor and push off into a squat position. Grab the inside of your ankles and use your elbows to push your knees out. Circle your hips.	Squat down. Grab your ankles. Use your elbows push your knees out. Circle your hips. Reverse.
Stand up and put your feet together. Bend your knees and put your hands on your knees and circle them in both directions. Slowly straighten your knees and at the last moment push them straight and let your feet slide back a few inches. Repeat three times.	Stand up. Feet together. Bend your knees. Circle round. Reverse. Bend and push straight. One. Two. Three.
Stand with your feet shoulders' width apart and put your hands on your hips and circle them in both directions. Then swing your hips from side to side.	Hands on your hips. Circle your hips. Reverse. Side to side.

Then with your hands on your hips roll your shoulders forward and backwards. Then raise them up and down.	Roll your shoulders forward. And backwards. Up and down.
Move the chin forward and back. Then down and back. Then look left and right. Then ear to each shoulder and make a half circle in front.	Chin in and out. Down and back. Looking left to right. Ear to shoulder. Half circles in front.
Close your fist and circle your arms in both directions.	Close your fists, circle your arms. Reverse.
Open your hands and open your arms with the palms up and cross your arms with the palms down. Then raise your arms up and down.	Open. Up and down.
Jump in place. Put your hands on your hips and cross your legs front and back. Then side to side. Then put your left leg forward and jump forward and back. Then side to side. Repeat on the opposite side.	Jumping. Hands on your hips, cross your feet front and back. Side to side. Left foot forward, forward and back. Side to side. Reverse. Forward and back. Side to side.
Jog in place. Take one step forward with your right foot, then one step forward with your left foot. Then take one step back with your right foot, then one step back with your left foot. Continue several times.	Jog in place. Forward-forward, back-back. Out-out, in-in. One-two, one-two.
Jump in place with your arms to your sides. Jump higher and then your highest, picking your knees up.	Jump. Jump a little higher. And your highest, pick up your knees.
Stop and adjust your uniform.	Yame. Turn around and adjust your gi if necessary.

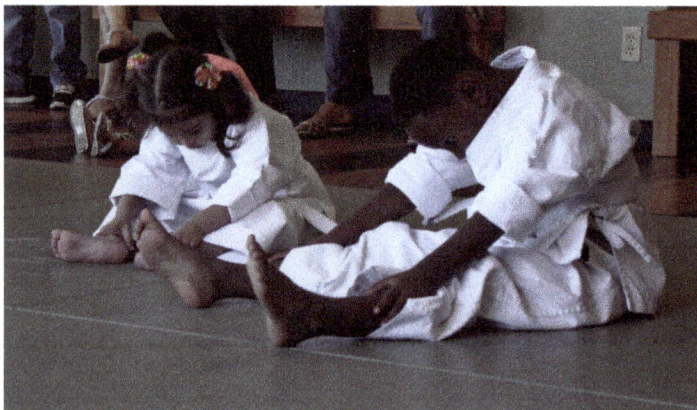

Basic Stretching

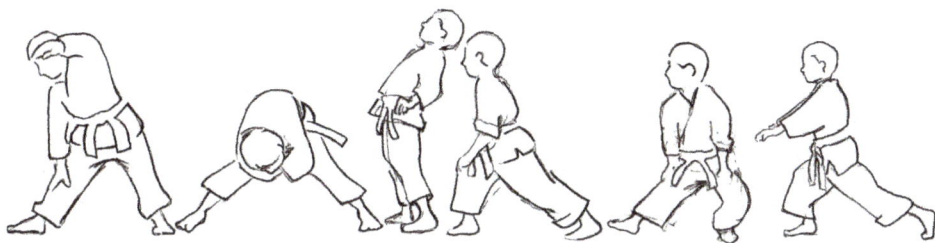

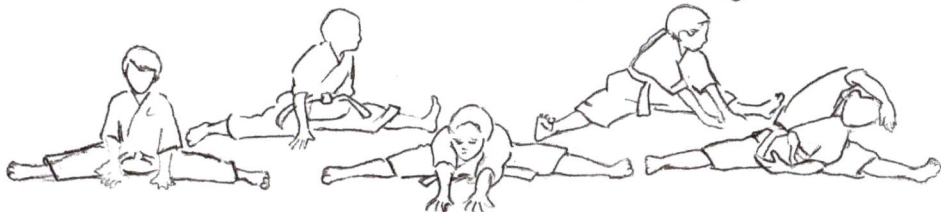

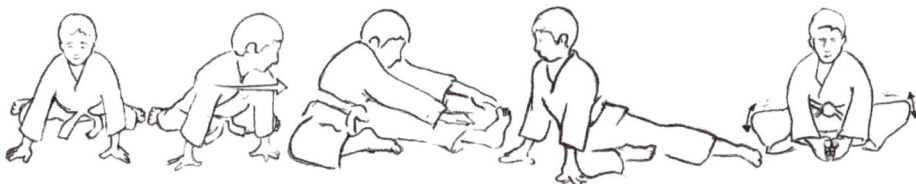

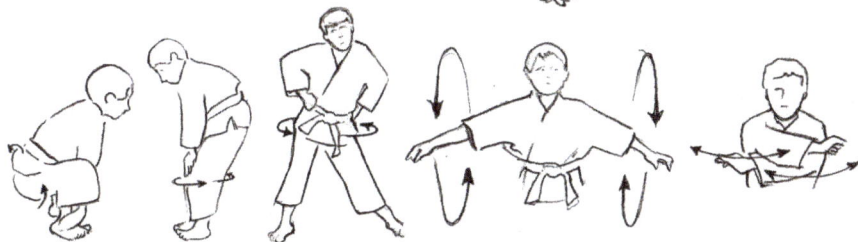

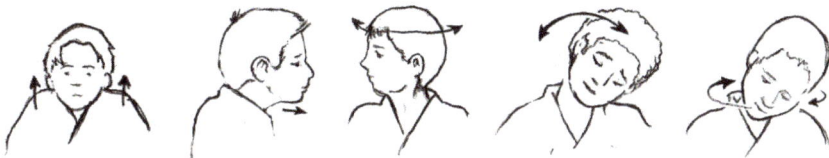

Basics/Kihon

Stances

Stances are stationary positions used both defensively and offensively; to provide support against a force coming towards you and a base to generate power from, whether attacking or counterattacking. During your beginning stage, you will learn three basic stances: side, forward, and back stance.

There are also three natural stances, all with your feet under your shoulders. One with your toes slightly turned out, a second with your toes straight, and a third with your toes slightly turned in. You will learn two feet together stances as well: One with your heels touching and your toes slightly turned out, and a second one with your heels and toes touching.

The body movements you will learn are vibration, rotation, and shifting. Shifting is the wide variety of ways you can move your body. This includes forward and back, side to side, up and down, and turning.

Techniques fall into four categories: thrusting, blocking, striking and kicking. This manual will describe two thrusting techniques – straight punch and spearhand; six blocking techniques – rising, outside forearm, down, sword hand, inside forearm and augmented; three striking techniques – hammer fist, side back fist and side elbow; and four kicking techniques – front snap, round house, side snap and side thrust.

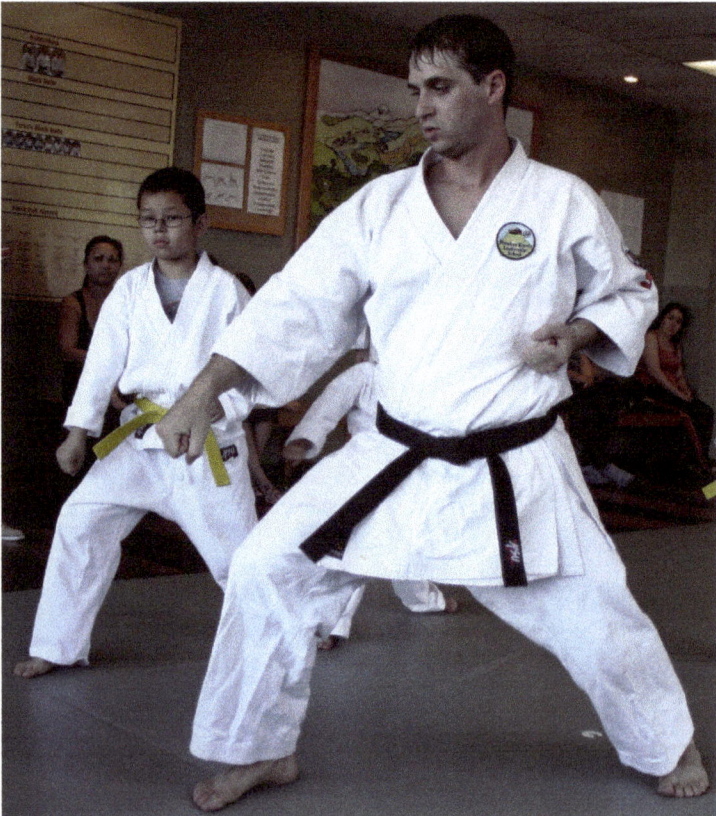

Forward Stance

Forward stance is the most useful of all the stances. It provides support when facing an opponent. This stance has two main hip positions – front-facing and half-front facing. In the front-facing position, the center of your body is facing straight forward. In the half-front facing position, the center of your body faces approximately 45 degrees to the side, pointing in the direction of your rear foot.

Length and Width

The length should be about twice the distance of your shoulders, measured from the heel of your rear foot to the heel of your front foot. The width should be one shoulder's length, measured from the inside of your front foot to the outside of your rear foot.

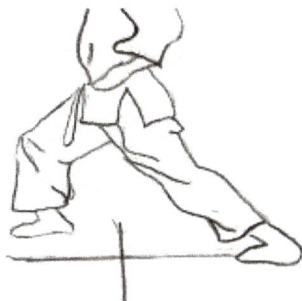

Foot Position

Turn your front foot slightly inside so the outside edge of your foot points straight forward, then turn your rear foot as far forward as you can. Ideally, it will point completely forward, but many beginners can only get it halfway.

Weight Distribution

Shift your weight so that 60% is on your front foot and 40% is on your rear foot. Bend your front knee over your big toe and slightly bend your back knee.

Leg Tension and Flow of Energy

The tension in your legs is what makes this stance dynamic. Your thighs are twisted either inward or outward, depending on which hip position you are in, while your feet remain stationary. In the front facing position, twist your upper legs inward, letting the energy that is created from this tension flow up your spine into your brain, making it alert and ready. Once your brain is fully activated, direct the flow of energy down the front of your body and into the floor, rooting yourself to the ground. Then start the flow of energy again to the outside, up, down and out. This is how you keep yourself fully energized.

If you're in the half-front facing position, twist your upper legs outward before directing the flow of energy upward.

Side Stance

Side stance supports your body by rooting your feet to the ground. It is also an excellent training stance.

Length and Width

There is no length to the side stance, because your feet are directly across from each other. The width of this stance is twice as wide as your shoulders.

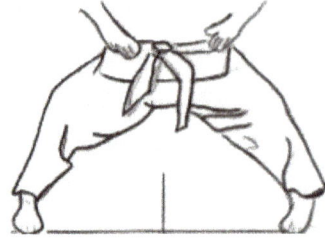

Foot Position

Turn both of your feet slightly inside so the outside edge of each foot points straight forward. Pretend you are standing in railroad tracks with your feet against the inside of the rails.

Weight Distribution

The weight distribution is 50/50, with your knees bent in the direction of your toes.

Leg Tension and Flow of Energy

Your thighs are twisted to the outside and the energy that is created is directed up the spine to the brain. Once your brain is fully activated, direct the flow of energy down the front of the body and into the floor rooting yourself to the ground.

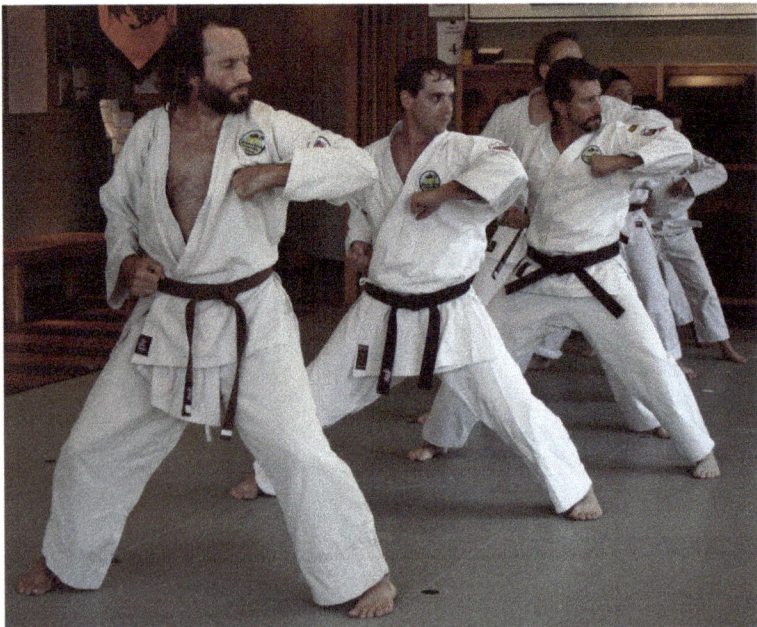

Back Stance

Back stance supports your body to the front with your weight distributed towards your back leg. It is very effective at giving the impression that you are further away than you actually are. You use this stance when you are close to an opponent. The body position is usually half-front facing, but can also be front facing.

Length and Width

The length is one and a half to two times the width of your shoulders, with your heels in a straight line.

Foot Position

Your front foot is turned slightly to the inside so the outside edge of the foot points straight forward. Your rear foot is turned 90 degrees to the side.

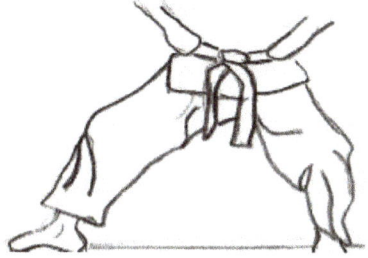

Weight Distribution

Your weight is distributed 70/30, with the rear knee deeply bent in the direction of your feet, with 70% of your weight on it. The front knee is slightly bent in the direction of the front foot. If your leg is locked straight and someone stomps on it or kicks it, the chances of getting a broken knee are very high.

Leg Tension and Flow of Energy

With your hips in the half-front facing body position, your thighs twist to the outside and the energy that is created is directed up the spine to the brain. Once your brain is fully activated, direct the flow of energy down the front of the body and into the floor rooting yourself to the ground.

Body Movement

Vibration

Body vibration is the action of turning one hip forward slightly, then the other side, and finally returning to your original position. You first learn body vibration while standing in natural or side stance. It is used to increase the speed of your techniques. It can be used to start or end a technique.

Rotation

Body rotation is when you move your hips from one position to another. It is most frequently used to move the hips from the half-front facing body position to the front-facing body position or vice versa. \|
You can use body rotation to bring more power to a technique, driving your punch or block with the torque of your hips.

Shifting

Shifting is the process of moving the body center, or hara, from its current position into another position. The body center is located at your waist level and in the center of your body. Some common ways to shift are stepping, sliding, half-stepping, cross-stepping, jumping, dropping, and a multitude of ways to turn.

Stepping

Stepping is exactly what it sounds like, stepping from one stance into another. Remember, when you're moving into a new stance with your leg, always swing it in close to your other foot and not in a straight line to your intended target. Swinging your foot in and out will actually create more speed than moving it in a straight line. Make sure the foot that is staying stationary is firmly rooted to the ground and your knees remain bent. You will have a more powerful technique if you simply move from stance to stance without straightening your legs. It takes valuable time and effort that could be better spent completing the move.

Sliding

Sliding can quickly move your body over a short distance. Your legs do not change positions while sliding. Simply lift your right foot, if you want to move to your right, or your front foot if you want to slide forward, and propel yourself with your left or rear leg. Your body will move quickly forward or sideways while staying parallel to the floor. Any upward movement will slow the process down and expose you to an attack, so stay close to the floor. A common problem is attempting to push your body forward before your lead foot is lifted off the floor. This results in a hop, which is by definition an upward movement.

Techniques

Thrusting

Thrusting techniques are techniques that use the end of the open hand or fist i.e. the fore knuckles of the fist in punching, the fingertips in the various spearhand techniques.

Straight Punch

The straight punch is the most common of all the thrusting techniques. It uses the fore knuckles of the index and middle fingers as a striking surface. Make your fist by rolling your fingers into the palm of your hand starting with the little finger and then placing the thumb across the index and middle fingers between your first and second knuckles (counting from the end of the finger).

Extend your left arm straight in front of you, with your fist at middle body level with your palm down. This is your draw hand arm and this position is the preparation for your draw hand. Your right arm is centered at the side of the body between the pelvis and the lower rib with your fist palm up. This arm is called the punching arm and it is in the draw hand position.

Now imagine a rope and a pulley mounted on the wall in front of you. One end of the rope is in the draw hand, the rope goes through the pulley and the other end is in the punching hand. Turn your draw hand over, then starts to pull it back to your hip.. Because your hands are connected by the rope, your punching hand will extend forward in the palm up position and twist over in the final two inches of the punch when you bring your draw hand to your hip. At the end of your punch, your body is contracted and all your energy is directed into an imaginary target about 4" in front of your fist.

Reverse Punch

A reverse punch is much like a straight punch, except it is used after another technique. With a step-in punch, your arms match your legs, while with a reverse punch you can have your left leg forward and punch with your right arm. Many counterattacks are reverse techniques, as they allow you to stay in place while stopping your opponent's attack.

Hook Punch

A hook punch curves across your body and is often used to stop attacks to your side. To perform a hook punch, start with your hand at your hip in the draw hand position. Bring your fist, still palm side up, forward and up, until your elbow is bent and your upper arm is parallel with the floor. Start to twist your arm over, and at the same time, bring your arm across your body. When you complete the punch, your fist should be palm side down and stopped at the opposite edge of your torso. Your arm should be tilted downwards at a slight angle, as if water could flow in a smooth line off your shoulder and down your fist to the floor.

Spearhand

The spearhand technique uses the tips of the index, middle, and ring fingers to thrust into a soft part of your opponent, such as their windpipe, solar plexus or between the ribs. Your hand is open, with your fingers straight and tightly held together.

The spearhand can be used in three different positions: the vertical spearhand, in which the thumb side of your open hand is up, the horizontal palm down position, and the horizontal palm up position. The vertical spearhand is the most common, and will often start from the open hand, palm up, draw hand position in front of the solar plexus. From here, turn your hand up slightly, and thrust your wrist forward.

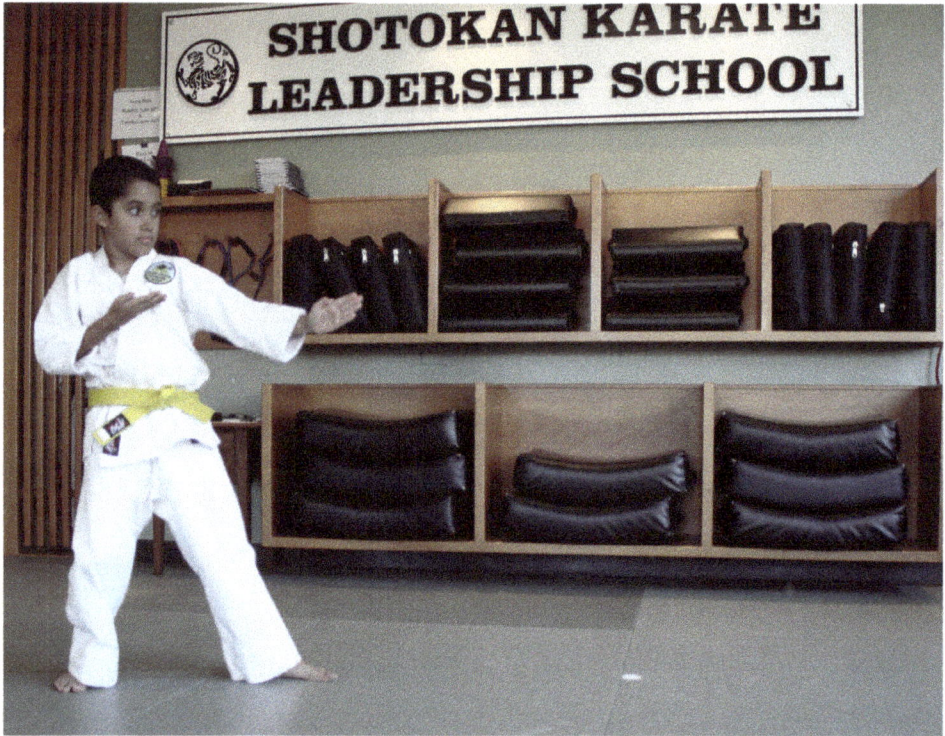

Striking

Striking techniques use the sides of the hand and the elbow. Unlike thrusting techniques, they will often use a circular motion to reach the target. The techniques presented here are only the simplest and most frequently used techniques. There are many others.

Hammer-fist Strike

The hammer-fist refers to the little finger side of the closed fist. In comparison to the knuckles, it is a soft surface and can be used effectively against hard parts of the opponent's body. The hammer-fist strike has several applications. The one you will learn as a beginner is the downward hammer-fist strike at your upper body level, particularly the collar bone, bridge of the nose, or the top of the head. Your arm starts down at your side and circles up, around, and downward to the target. Use your shoulder as the center of the circle. If the collar bone is your target, your arm should finish the technique extended straight out from your shoulder with your elbow slightly bent, and the hammer-fist side of your fist facing downward.

Side Backfist Strike

The side backfist strike uses the top of the first knuckles of the index and middle fingers as the striking surface.

The technique can be used with a whipping or thrusting motion. To achieve a whipping motion, your fist will hit the target and immediately snap back. To use a thrusting motion, your fist will penetrate the target and your arm will lock in position before the technique is drawn back.

The most common way of executing the technique starts with your fist at chest level, the palm side facing downwards and your elbow pointing towards the target. Whip your arm out and back to your chest. Just before making contact with the target, turn your fist over so the thumb side of your fist is up and the back of your fist comes in contact with the side of the target.

The second most common way of executing the technique starts with your hand at the opposite hip, the thumb side up and the elbow pointed at the target. Thrust your hand to the target and lock it in position. Use the back of your fist to hit the target.

Side Elbow Strike

The side elbow strike is one of the most powerful techniques in Shotokan karate. Start with your arm across your body and parallel to the floor. Your fist should be in the thumb up position. Move your arm straight to the side until your forearm is parallel to the line of your toes. Twist your arm inward and stop with the back of your hand up. The tip of your elbow is the striking surface.

Blocking

Blocks make up the majority of karate's techniques. You can block with your arms and your legs, but the most common blocks use your arms: rising, outside forearm, down, and sword hand. The primary purpose of blocking is to break your opponent's concentration long enough to execute an effective counterattack. Things to watch for when blocking include the striking surface, the course, and angle of your arm upon completion.

Some blocks require a single step and others two steps. These will be referred to as the preparation stage and the execution stage.

Rising Block

The rising block requires only a single motion. Start the rising block from your draw hand at your hip. Use your arm to cut a diagonal course across the front of your body, then straight up with the palm side of your fist facing towards your body. Your arm then follows a very gradual circular course towards the back. When your arm is about the level of your forehead, twist your wrist over so the palm side if your fist is

Shotokan Karate

facing away from your body. In the final position, your arm is at a 45-degree angle, with your elbow about one fist distance from the corner of your forehead.

Outside Forearm Block

The outside forearm block can be completed in two steps. Bring your fist up to your left ear with your palm facing forwards, your elbow out to your side, and your upper arm parallel to the floor. From this position, start a circular course with your bent arm towards the front of your body, bringing your elbow within a fist's distance of your body. Your arm should be bent in a 45-degree angle, with your fist across from your shoulder.

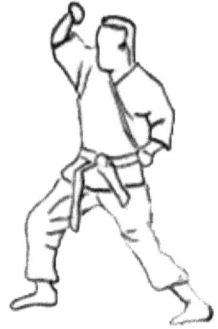

Down Block

The down block requires a two-stage process as well. Bring your blocking arm up to your opposite shoulder with your little finger touching your collar bone and your elbow close to your body. When the preparation is complete, bring your arm down the front of your body and stop it with the outside edge of your arm in alignment with the outside edge of your body.

During the downward motion, your elbow is held close to your body. At the end of the movement, your elbow is approximately one fist distance from your body. As you complete the movement, twist your arm so the little finger side of your fist is turned outwards. When the block is complete, the little finger side of your fist is facing outwards.

Sword Hand Block

Make a sword hand block by opening your hand and holding your fingers straight and tightly together. The outside edge of your palm is the blocking surface. Your arm is bent at the elbow, but not at the wrist.

The sword hand block requires two steps. Bring your hand, palm open, to your opposite shoulder, just like you did to prepare for the down block. To execute the block, move your arm diagonally across your body, your hand remaining at shoulder height. In the final position, the little finger edge of your arm is even with the side of your body and perpendicular to the floor. Your forearm is at an approximately 45-degree angle with your body, while your elbow is one fist distance from the side of your body.

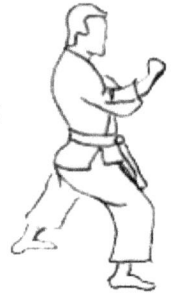

Inside Forearm Block

The inside forearm block starts from underneath the opposite arm and finishes in the same position as the outside forearm block, perpendicular to the floor with your elbow about one fist distance from your body, and your arm bent at about a 45 degree angle. Your fist is about the same height as your shoulders. The difference between the two blocks is that the inside forearm block starts from across the body and uses the thumb edge of your

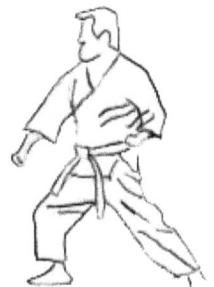

hand to block, and the outside forearm block starts near your ear and uses the little finger edge of your forearm to block.

After positioning your blocking arm under the opposite arm close to your armpit, pull your arm out from under it while keeping your elbow close to your body. Turn your arm over so that the blocking surface comes in contact with the attacker's arm.

Augmented Block

Augment means "to help." One hand supports and helps the other one in this block. An inside forearm block is made with one arm, with the other fist is against your elbow, the palm side of your fist facing up.

To execute a right augmented block, take your right fist and place it near your left shoulder, while holding your right elbow close to your body. At the same time, place your left fist near your right elbow with your palm down. Quickly bring your right forearm over into an outside forearm block and twist your left fist over so it faces palm up and rests tightly against your right elbow.

Kicking

Kicking techniques primarily use your foot as the striking surface, but other parts of your leg can be used as well. Kicks are either snapping or thrusting movements, and are considered to be the most powerful techniques in karate. Snapping is a whip-like motion, with your lower leg moving out and back. A critical factor in the success of any snap kick is the positioning of your knee. Only after you have snapped your leg out and back can your knee position change. The power of your technique comes from hitting the target and pulling back before the impact can ricochet back into the body. Thrusting is like a battering ram; your leg is extended, locked straight, brought back to your body and then the floor. The power of this kick comes from locking your leg at the end.

Front Snap Kick

The front snap kick uses the ball of your foot as the striking surface, and a whipping motion to reach the target. Start by raising your kicking leg as high as you can, while flexing your toes and pressing the ball of your foot forward. Extend your lower leg out while extending your ankle, so the ball of your foot reaches maximum extension and height. The faster the whipping motion, the more powerful the kick. Your target is centered in front of you and perpendicular to the floor.

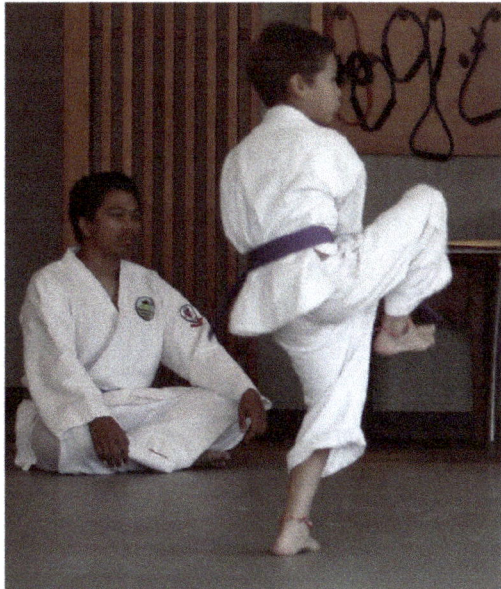

Roundhouse Kick

The roundhouse kick utilizes your entire foot as a striking surface, and derives power from the twisting motion of your hips. Start by lifting your knee out to the side, your leg bent and parallel to the ground. Twist your body from your hips so your leg is facing the front, then snap your leg out and back. Step down in a forward stance.

Side Snap Kick

To perform a right side snap kick, stand in side stance and turn your head to the right. Staying low in your stance, cross your left foot over your right. Keep your feet close together, and your right foot flat on the floor. Shift your weight onto your left leg, planting your foot on the ground as you lift your right leg up. Snap your right leg out and back before stepping down into a side stance.

Side Thrust Kick

A side thrust kick is performed much like a side snap kick, except for the execution of the kick. Instead of snapping your leg out and back, turn your hips over and lock your leg in place. After completing the kick, bring your leg back and down.

Kumite/Sparring

Sparring will teach you how to use and apply the basics you will learn. It is also excellent practice for defense situations outside the school. Shotokan Karate Leadership School® practices non-contact sparring, which means that when students practice, they don't hit each other. For students who are in excellent physical condition and higher ranking, more contact can be made, but usually only during free sparring. Both students must agree to the level of contact.

There are four levels of sparring: multi-step, one-step, semi-free and free. Beginners start with multi-step sparring, usually this is three-step sparring.

Multi-step

There are three learning points for multi-step sparring. First, your techniques must be effective. This means the your technique must actually work – it can't be wimpy. The work that your technique must do is to stop your opponent. Every technique does that in a slightly different way. The basic elements of each technique are correct form, speed and the stopping power created from contracting your muscles thoroughly known as kime. Without an effective technique, you cannot stop your opponent, which is the goal of self-defense. If you had a hammer and every time you tried to pound a nail, the head came off; it wouldn't be much of a hammer. Your hammer would not be effective. The same is true for your technique. You have to know your technique will be useful.

Second, you must be able to execute your technique while in motion. It's one thing to have a good technique while you're standing still, and another thing to have a good technique while you're moving.

Third, you must coordinate these two things with your breathing. Controlling your breath is the secret to controlling your mind. If you lose control of your breath, you can easily go into a state of panic and function ineffectively. With controlled breathing, you can remain calm and allow yourself to function well in a stressful or dangerous situation.

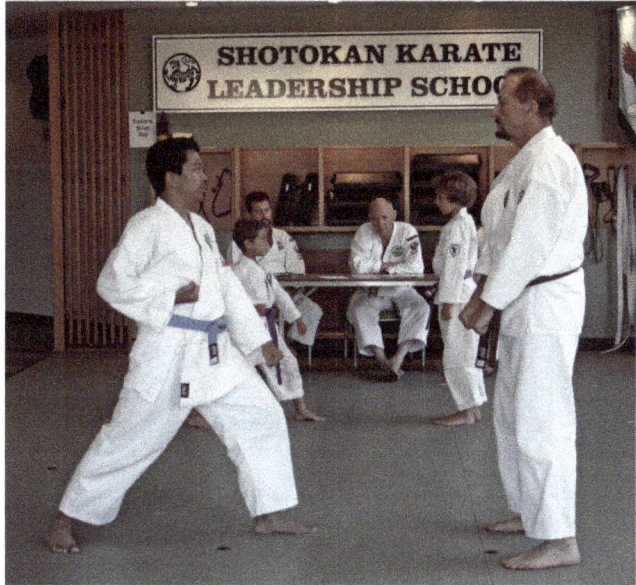

A sample sequence is described below:

Both students stand at bowing distance and bow to one another. The bowing distance is approximately kicking distance. Specifically, take one step forward with one leg and perform a front kick with your rear leg. The person with shorter legs will stand farther back than the person with longer legs, because the person with longer legs can reach farther.

Bow with your heels together and your toes open. Stand upright and look directly into the left eye of the other person. Then bend your upper body at the hips to about a 45-degree angle, while keeping your back straight. Lower your eyes to your partner's lower body or feet as you bow. Straighten up and look directly into the left eye of your partner. This should take about 3 seconds to complete. Left is considered receiving and right is considered giving so looking into your opponent's left eye means that he or she must receive you.

At this point, the designated defender moves to within striking distance. Striking distance is the distance that the attacker could actually hit the defender with a step-in punch and penetrate by 2-4 inches. This distance can be judged by having the attacker perform a slow-motion step-in punch directed to a point over the left shoulder of the defender. When the attacker actually attacks, his or her technique will be directed towards the opponent's chin or throat for an upper body attack, to their solar plexus for a middle body attack and to a point directly above their belt for a lower body punch.

Once the defender is within striking distance, the attacker will announce in a serious voice the technique they will use and the target they are aiming for. We use Japanese terminology for this. A step-in punch to the upper body is announced as 'oizuki jodan,' and a step-in punch to the middle body is 'oizuki chudan.' After announcing the technique and target, the attacker will wait for the count, then attack, or wait until opponent has breathed out before attacking.

The attacker's first attack is with their right arm and is directed to the defender's upper body. The defender will step back with his or her right leg and perform the first rising block with their left arm. The attacker will continue with the next two attacks while the defender steps back and performs rising blocks. After the third rising block, the defender counterattacks to the attacker's middle body with a right reverse punch. When the counterattack is finished, both students return to natural stance. The attacker steps backwards and the defender steps forward. The roles are then reversed, with the defender becoming the attacker and the attacker becoming the defender. Upon completion of the upper body attacks, the sequence starts over with the first student attacking the middle body three times, followed by the second student attacking the middle body three times.

One-step

Once a student has reached green belt, they are taught and tested on one-step sparring. The three learning points of one-step sparring are: timing, distancing, and an effective counterattack.

The first learning point, timing, is vital in sparring. It is important to watch your opponent and attack when they are breathing out and more relaxed. If you are defending yourself, make sure you are watching your opponent carefully and are not caught off guard.

The second learning point, distancing, is just as important as timing. If you have an excellent technique, but cannot reach your opponent, it is useless. If you need, practice punch over your opponent's shoulder to make sure your punch can penetrate them by 2 to 4 inches. Let them know what you're doing ahead of time, however. You do not want to accidentally punch them in the face.

The last learning point of one-step sparring is certainly not least. An effective counterattack is just as important as an effective block or attack. If you can block your opponent, but not prevent them from attacking you again, your blocks will only do you so much good.

An example of one-step sparring is explained below:

Both students start at the same distance as multi-step sparring. The defender steps forward one stance length, then the attacker steps within striking distance. It is vitally important to make sure that you have set your distance properly at this stage. The attacker steps back with their right leg, into the left down block position, and announces 'oizuki jodan.' The attacker then proceeds to attack. The defender steps back with their right leg, and performs a rising block with their left arm. The defender counterattacks to the middle body. Both the defender and attacker step back into natural stance. The attacker switches his or her legs and attacks again, this time with their left arm. The defender steps back and blocks with their right arm, then counterattacks to the middle body again. The process is repeated once more, this time to the middle body. The attacker attacks twice, once with their right leg forward and once with their left leg forward.

Once the attacker has attacked a total of four times, the students change roles and the defender is now the attacker. Repeat the process, attacking twice to the upper body and twice to the middle body for a total of four attacks. Once the students are finished, they should return to their starting positions and bow to each other.

When students reach 4th kyu purple belt, they will learn to use kicking in addition to punching, in one-step sparring. There are two possible attacks: 'Mae geri chudan,' front snap kicking to the middle body, and 'yoko kekomi chudan,' side thrust kicking to the middle body. The sequence of events is the same as the step-in punch attacks, except for the blocking techniques. The front snap kick is blocked with a down block to the thigh, while the side thrust kick is side-stepped so the attacker lands in side stance with his or her back facing the defender. The defender's counterattack is to the attacker's spine or kidneys.

Semi-free

The three learning points of semi-free sparring are: See and take advantage of an opening, catch your opponent in one step, and block and counter in one breath.

The first learning point is vital to catching your opponent off-guard. It's best to wait as long as possible before attacking. Let your opponent become relaxed and let their guard down. Wait for them to breathe in, and watch carefully to see if their balance is off or anything is amiss. As soon as you see the opening, attack. Speed is not as important as accuracy. Practice taking advantage of openings, and as you get better, you will also get faster.

Catching your opponent in one step requires that you set the proper distance before you attack. Make sure you know how far from your opponent you have to be in order to reach them in one step. Remember that your attack should penetrate by two to four inches and be prepared to shift in if they step back faster than you can reach them.

Blocking and countering in one breath will give you more power and the speed needed to protect yourself. In a real life-or-death situation, you must be conscious of your breathing, because if you let it become fast or panicked, you will lose control of yourself and your brain will switch into panic mode.

Free

There are also three major learning points for free sparring. They are… create openings, lead your opponent to a position favorable to you, and use various and changing techniques. The end result of free sparring is that you have stopped your opponent.

Free sparring, is best begun by assuming free stance outside of striking distance while you take a moment to assess the strengths and weaknesses of your opponent in relation to your strengths and weaknesses. After assessing your opponent you will then form an initial strategy as to how you are going to stop this opponent.

In assessing your opponent don't forget to apply what you've learned from the study of personality traits as they relate to our four houses: Kraken (water), Terra (earth), Fire Dragon (fire), and Sora (air). Ask yourself, for example, 'What would a person who is predominately a water element be like and how would they likely attack and defend?' Once you've done that you're now ready to begin to implement your strategy. Keep in mind though that the situation could change at any moment, and that you will have to adjust your plans accordingly.

There are three types of free sparring: dojo sparring, tournament sparring, and actual combat. Dojo sparring is a free exchange between two people who are working together to improve each other's techniques, tactics and strategies. Tournament sparring is a match wherein the contestants are attempting to score points while the match is overseen by a referee, who controls the match, and awards points. Actual combat is a real fight. We are preparing ourselves to do well in an actual fight but we cannot practice this without the risk of serious injury and all the negative emotion that comes with it.

Specialized Self-Defense

You will practice specialized self-defense from time to time in class. There will be contact made and gentler practice of throws and grabs. It is important to be careful while practicing with fellow students, because these moves do work and you can cause serious injury or pain. Tap out if you need, and pay attention to see if your partner is tapping out. A tap out is two quick taps or slaps on the ground, your body, or your opponent's body. Make sure that you pull yourself back before completing the move, or if you have to go through with it, do it gently, and check with your partner that they are okay with what you're doing.

Some of the kinds of self-defense you will learn are: against grabs, multiple opponents, from the floor, from a chair. You will also learn how to protect yourself from attacks with sticks and knives, with your hands tied, and much more.

Kata/Forms

Kata is a series of movements against imaginary opponents. It is a wonderful way to practice because it uses your imagination – your most powerful weapon. Self-defense works similarly. You can imagine being attacked; then devise ways to stop the attack. Or, you could be attacked and get away, but don't like what you did, and devise a better way. You could also develop your techniques; then create ways to use those techniques.

Kata is the lifeblood of karate. Karate is renewed and invigorated each time it is performed properly. It is an art that has been around for thousands of years, and it will continue for thousands of years because kata develops and trains your imagination. Albert Einstein said, "Imagination is more important than knowledge. For knowledge is limited to all we now know and understand, while imagination embraces the entire world, and all there ever will be to know and understand." Your ability to dream is tied to your imagination, and it is through your dreams that new life can be discovered.

The Heian Katas

The first kata you will learn is Heian Shodan, or Heian 1. 'Heian' means peace, and 'shodan' means first step or first level. There are 5 katas in the Heian group. The other 4 katas in this group are named Heian Nidan (2), Heian Sandan (3), Heian Yondan (4) and Heian Godan (5).

Heian Shodan

Heian Shodan has 21 movements that are used against eight imaginary opponents.

Start from the feet together position, with your toes open, and bow. Move into natural stance by stepping your right leg ½ shoulder's width to the right and then stepping your left leg ½ shoulder's width to the left.

1. Turn 90 degrees to the left; step into a left forward stance and down block.
2. Perform a right step-in punch middle body level.
3. Turn right 180 degrees to the rear by moving the right front leg around to the back and perform a down block with your right arm.
4. Pull your front foot halfway back, circle your right arm at the shoulder, and strike at the collarbone level with a right hammer fist strike.
5. Perform a left step-in punch middle body level.
6. Turn 90 degrees to the left; step into a left forward stance and down block you're your left arm.
7. As you begin to step forward into a right forward stance raise your left hand up to the rising block position with your hand in the sword hand position. Finish the step forward and perform a right rising block.
8. As you begin to step forward into a left forward stance open your right hand to the sword hand position. Finish the step forward and perform a left rising block.
9. As you begin to step forward into a right forward stance open your left hand to

the sword hand position. Finish the step forward and perform a right rising block. Kiai.

10. Pivot backwards on your right foot 270 degrees; turn to your right side; step into a left forward stance and perform a left down block.
11. Perform a right step-in punch middle body level.
12. Turn right 180 degrees to the rear by moving the right front leg around to the back and perform a down block with your right arm.
13. Perform a left step-in punch middle body level.
14. Turn 90 degrees to the left; step into a left forward stance and down block you're your left arm.
15. Perform a right step-in punch middle body level.
16. Perform a left step-in punch middle body level.
17. Perform a right step-in punch middle body level. Kiai.
18. Pivot backwards on your right foot 270 degrees; turn to your right side; step into a left back stance and perform a left sword hand block.
19. Step diagonally forward to the right into right back stance and perform a right sword hand block.
20. Turn 135 degrees to the right; step into a right back stance; and perform a right sword hand block.
21. Step diagonally forward to the left into left back stance and perform a left sword hand block.

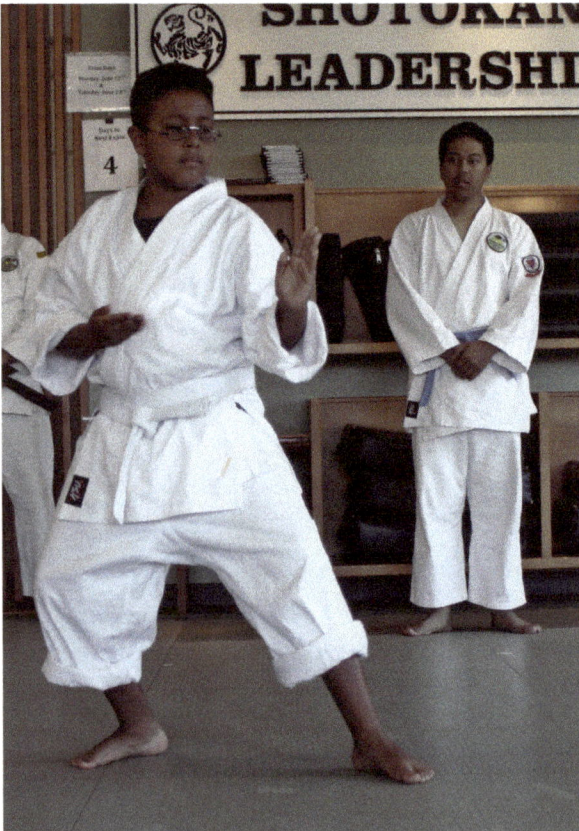

Withdraw your left leg, return to natural stance and demonstrate zanshin – remaining mind. Move your left leg halfway towards your right leg and then your right leg halfway towards your left leg into the feet together, toes open, stance and bow.

Heian Shodan

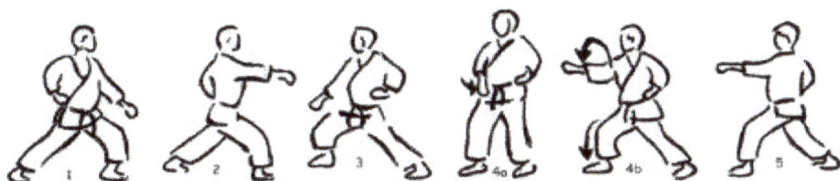

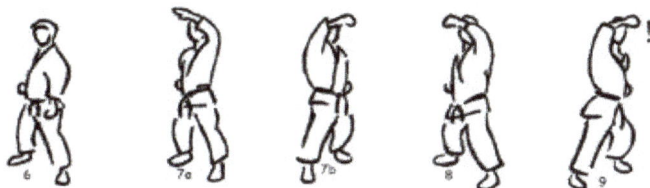

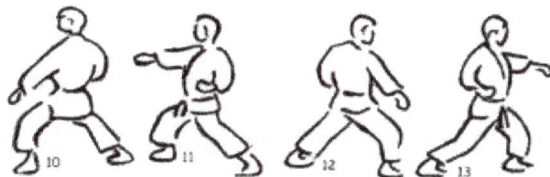

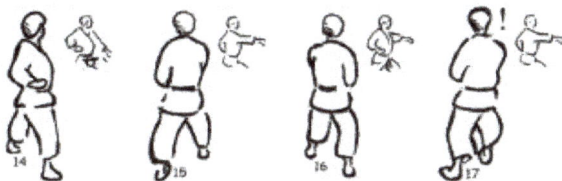

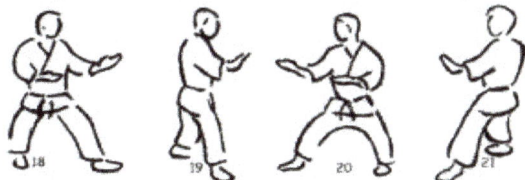

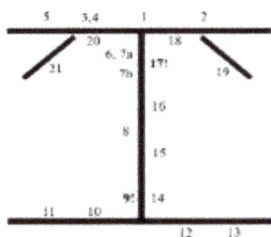

61

Heian Nidan

Heian Nidan has 26 movements that are used against twelve imaginary opponents.

Start from the feet together position, with your toes open, and bow. Move into natural stance by stepping your right leg ½ shoulder's width to the right and then stepping your left leg ½ shoulder's width to the left.

1. Turn 90° to the left, stepping out with your left leg into back stance. Perform an upper level inside forearm block using the back of the forearm with your left arm, and a rising block to the front with your right arm.
2. Sweep your left arm to your right shoulder, little finger side of your fist against your collarbone. With your right arm, execute an outside forearm block to the left.
3. Punch with your left hand to your left, and pull your right hand to your hip in the draw hand position.
4. Pivot to your right, moving your feet into a right back stance, but keeping them on the ground. Perform a right upper level inside forearm block using the back of the forearm, and with the left arm perform a rising block to the front.
5. Sweep your right arm to your left shoulder, and execute an outside forearm motion to the right with your left arm.
6. Punch with your right hand to your right, and pull your left hand to your hip in the draw hand position.
7. Turn your head and look to the rear while drawing the left foot 30% of the way forward to the right foot, or just under your body. You are positioning it to be the stance leg of a side snap kick to the rear. At the same time, stack your right fist on top of your left draw hand, with the little finger side of your fist in contact with the folded fingers of your draw hand. Pick up your right leg with your knee turned 45 degrees to the back, with the right kicking foot near the knee of your left stance leg. Perform a right side snap kick and a side backfist strike to the rear.
8. After side snap kicking, look to the front, position your left open hand at your right shoulder and extend your right open hand to the front, then step back with your right leg into back stance and execute a left sword hand block.
9. Step forward and execute a right back stance sword hand block.
10. Step forward and execute a left back stance sword hand block.
11. Step forward and perform a pressing block with your left hand, while leaving your left elbow in place. Snap your hand downward to a position parallel to the floor. At the same time, execute a spearhand thrust with your right hand. In the final position, the elbow of your right spearhand will rest on top of the wrist of the left pressing block. Kiai.
12. Pivot on your right foot 270° backwards, turning to your right, and step into a left back stance and left sword hand block.
13. Step diagonally forward and to the right, into right back stance and right sword hand block.
14. Turn right 135° to the rear while withdrawing the right leg and stepping forward into right back stance and right sword hand block.
15. Step diagonally forward and to the left, into left back stance and left sword hand block.

16. Look 22 ½° back to the left. Twist your hips to a reverse front-facing position to the rear. Step your left leg across in preparation for a left forward stance, extend your left hand and reach your right hand from the draw hand position in front of the solar plexus to under the left arm. Using body vibration, pull your right arm out from under your left arm and perform a right reverse inside forearm block.
17. Perform a front snap kick with your right leg.
18. After kicking, step forward into a right forward stance and perform a left reverse punch.
19. While rotating your hips to a reverse front facing position, put your left arm under your right arm and perform a left inside forearm block.
20. Perform a front snap kick with your left leg.
21. After kicking, step forward into a left forward stance and perform a right reverse punch.
22. Continue with another step towards the rear and perform a right augmented block.
23. Pivot on your right foot 270° backwards, turning to your right, and step into a left inline forward stance and execute a left down block.
24. Step diagonally forward and to the right into a right forward stance and perform a right rising block.
25. Turn 135 degrees to the right, step into a right inline forward stance and execute a right down block.
26. Step diagonally forward and to the left into a left forward stance and perform a left rising block.

Withdraw your left leg, return to natural stance and demonstrate zanshin – remaining mind. Move your left leg halfway towards your right leg, then your right leg halfway towards your left leg into the feet together, toes open stance, and bow.

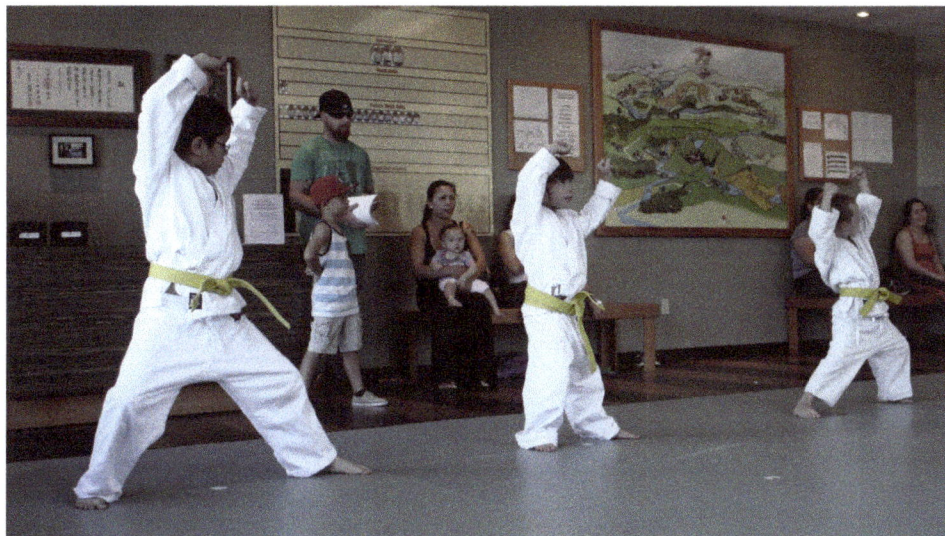

Heian Nidan

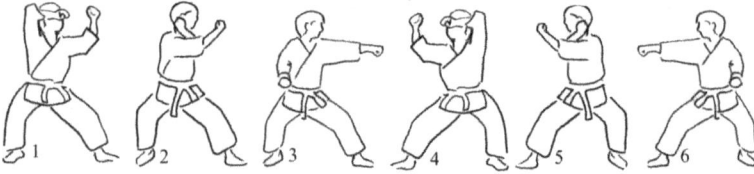

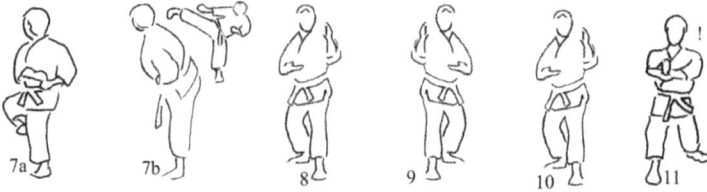

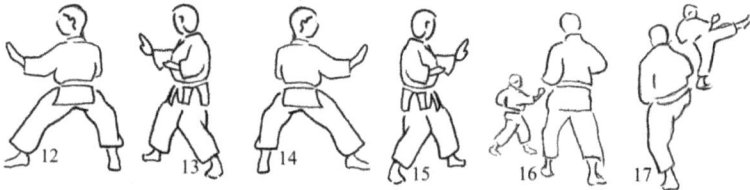

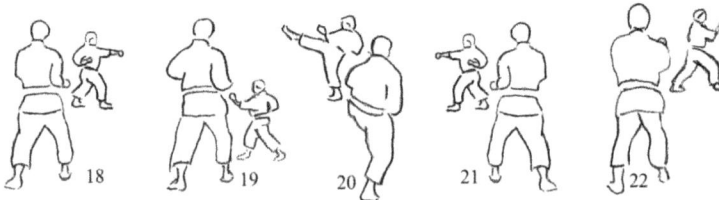

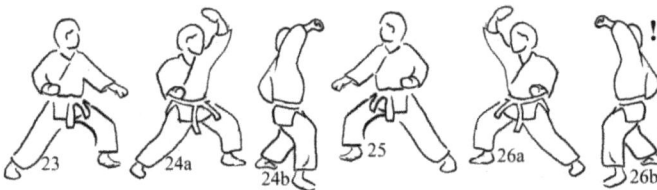

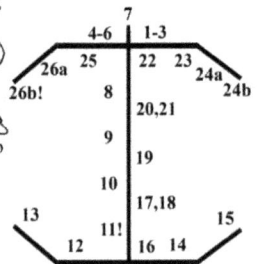

Heian Sandan

Heian Sandan has 20 movements that are used against imaginary opponents.

Start from the feet together position, with your toes open, and bow. Move into natural stance by stepping your right leg ½ shoulder's width to the right and then stepping your left leg ½ shoulder's width to the left.

1. Turn 90° to the left, stepping out with your left leg into back stance. Perform a left inside forearm block to the middle body.
2. Stand up in the feet together position, performing an inside forearm block with your right arm, making sure your elbows cross. Your left hand should be in a down block.
3. Execute a left inside forearm block, again making sure your elbows cross. Your right hand should be in a down block.
4. Turn 180° to your right, stepping out with your right leg into back stance. Perform a right inside forearm block.
5. Stand up in the feet together position and perform a left inside forearm block and a right down block.
6. Execute a right inside forearm block, again making sure your elbows cross. Your left hand should be in a down block.
7. Turn 90° to your left and face the front, stepping out into a left back stance and executing a left augmented block.
8. Step forward into a right forward stance and perform a right spearhand attack and left pressing block.
9. Turn your right hand over as you turn to your right 180° and land in side stance. Perform a side backfist strike to the middle body. Your head should be facing the front and your feet should be facing the side of the room.
10. Step-in punch to the middle body with your right leg and your right arm. Kiai.
11. Turn your left foot around so it faces the back of the room and stand up in the feet together position, facing the back of the room. Your hands should be in fists and rest on top of your hips with your elbows pointing to the sides. This is a slow movement.
12. Pick up your right foot as high as you can and land in a side stance. Use your elbow to block, tilting it forwards as you land.
13. Use body vibration to whip your right arm out and back in a backfist strike across from your collarbone.
14. Turn your right foot 90° so it faces forward, then lift your left foot as high as you can while pivoting on your right. You should land in another side stance and perform an elbow block again, this time with your left arm.
15. Use body vibration to whip your left arm out and back in a backfist strike across from your collarbone.
16. Turn your left foot 90° so it faces forward; then lift your right foot as high as you can while pivoting on your left. You should land in side stance and perform an elbow block again, this time with your right arm.
17. Use body vibration to whip your right arm out and back in a backfist strike across from your collarbone.
18. This movement is usually broken down into two parts. For the first part, shift your stance to an inline forward stance. Your left hand at your hip should change into a normal draw hand and your right hand should be extended

forward, palm open and facing away from you, at a 90° angle with your wrist. For the second part, step-in punch with your left arm and leg.

19. Bring your right foot up under your shoulders and swing it out so you are in a crude approximation of side stance. Pivot on your right foot, turning behind and to your left. You should land in a side stance facing the front of the room. At the same time, punch over your left shoulder with your right arm. Your left arm is in the draw hand position at your hip.

20. Pick your right foot up and shift to your right, remaining in side stance. At the same time, punch over your right shoulder with your left arm and bring your right hand to the draw hand position. Kiai.

Withdraw your right leg, return to natural stance and demonstrate zanshin – remaining mind. Move your left leg halfway towards your right leg, then your right leg halfway towards your left leg into the feet together, toes open stance, and bow.

Heian Yondan

Start from the feet together position, with your toes open, and bow. Move into natural stance by stepping your right leg ½ shoulder's width to the right and then stepping your left leg ½ shoulder's width to the left.

1. Turn 90° to your left; slowly step into a left back stance and perform a left upper level open handed forearm block; and a right open-handed rising block to the front.
2. Slowly pivot 180° to your right and change into a right back stance while performing a right upper level open-handed forearm block and a left open-handed rising block to the front.
3. Turn 90° to the front; step into a left forward stance and perform a lower level X block with your right wrist on top of your left.
4. Step forward into a right back stance and execute a right augmented block.
5. Turn your head 90° to the left; pick up your left leg and position it for the start of a side snap kick to the left while stacking your left hand on your right draw-hand.
6. Simultaneously perform a left backfist strike and a left side snap kick.
7. Step into a left forward stance and execute a forward elbow strike with your left arm.
8. Bring your left leg under your body while turning 180° to the right; pick up your right leg and position it for a right side snap kick while stacking your right hand on top of your left draw hand.
9. Simultaneously perform a right backfist strike and a right side snap kick.
10. Step into a right forward stance and execute a forward elbow strike with your right arm.
11. While pivoting on both feet 90° to the left into a left forward stance; circle your left sword hand down in front of your body and up to the rising block position. At the same time circle your right sword hand up to the rising block position and then to an upper level outside sword hand strike.
12. Perform a right front snap kick.
13. Leap forward 1 ½ stance distance into a right cross-footed stance and perform a right downward backfist strike to the front. Kiai.
14. Slowly pivot on your right foot 270 degrees to the rear; step into a left back stance while performing a reverse wedge block.
15. Perform a right front snap kick.
16. Step into a right forward stance and perform a right step-in punch to the middle body.
17. Perform a left reverse punch to the middle body.
18. Pivot 90° to the right and slowly step into a right back stance and perform a reverse wedge block.
19. Front snap kick with your left leg.
20. Step into a left forward stance and perform a left step-in punch to the middle body.
21. Perform a right reverse punch to the middle body.
22. Pivot 45° to the left on your right rear leg; step into a left back stance and perform a left augmented block.
23. Step forward into right back stance and perform a right augmented block.
24. Step forward into left back stance and perform a left augmented block.

25. Shift your weight onto your left leg while extending both hands out at upper body level in the sword hand position; then perform a right upper level knee kick while bringing both hands down to the side of your right knee and closing your fists. Kiai.
26. Then pivot 180° on your left leg, turn to the front, and step to the back into a left back stance while performing a left sword hand block.
27. Step forward in a right back stance and perform a right sword hand block.

Withdraw your right leg, return to natural stance and demonstrate zanshin – remaining mind. Move your left leg halfway towards your right leg, then your right leg halfway towards your left leg into the feet together, toes open stance, and bow.

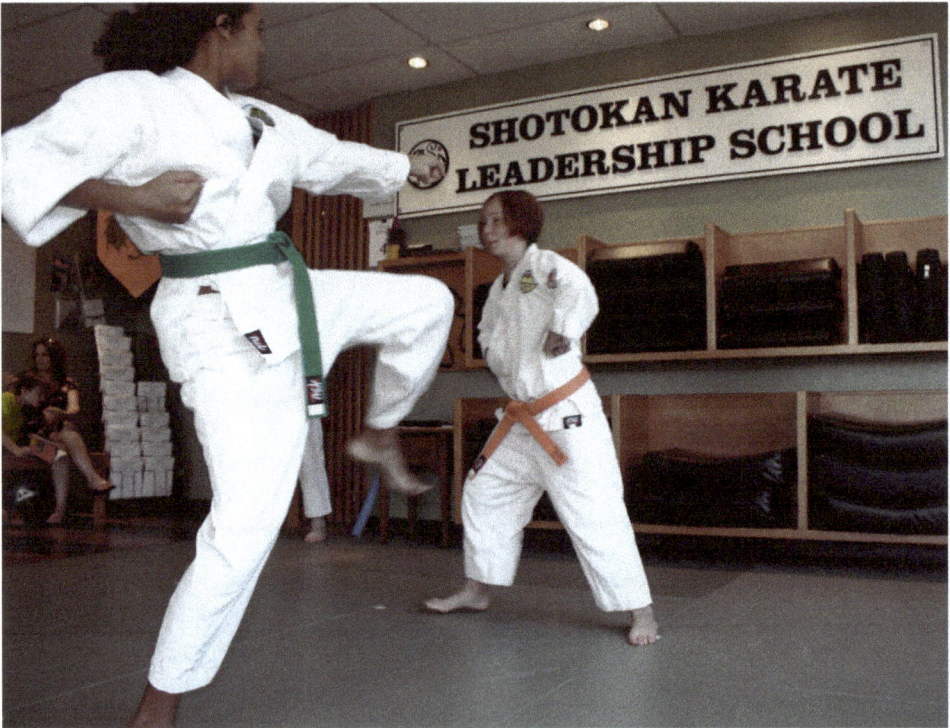

Heian Godan

Start from the feet together position, with your toes open, and bow. Move into natural stance by stepping your right leg ½ shoulder's width to the right and then stepping your left leg ½ shoulder's width to the left.

1. Turn 90° to the left, step out with your left leg into back stance. Perform a left inside forearm block to the middle body.
2. Perform a right reverse punch to the middle body.
3. Turn 180° to the right; pivot on your left foot and slowly draw your right foot to your left foot and stand in the feet together position while performing a left hook punch to the middle body.
4. Drop your weight and step into a right back stance while performing a right inside forearm block.
5. Perform a left reverse punch to the middle body.
6. Turn 90° to the left and pivot on your right foot while slowly drawing your left foot over to your right foot; stand up in the feet together position. At the same time, perform a right hook punch to the middle body.
7. Step forward into a right back stance and execute a right augmented block.
8. Step into a left forward stance and perform a lower level X block with your right wrist on top of your left.
9. Perform an open-handed upper level X block.
10. Press your left palm down onto your right palm and position your hands in a left pressing block position.
11. Begin to step forward with your right leg and perform a left side hammer-fist strike.
12. Complete the step forward and perform a right step-in punch to the middle body. Kiai.
13. Leaving your front foot in place and pivot 180° to the rear and perform a right down block.
14. Turn your head 180° back to the front and perform a vertical sword hand block and immediately change it into a backhand block.
15. Perform a right crescent kick to your left hand.
16. Step into side stance and perform a right forward elbow strike to your left hand.
17. Pivot 90° to your right; step into a right cross-footed stance and perform a right augmented block.
18. Pivot 180° to the rear; step into a V stance and perform a right upper level close punch with your left arm in a cover position in front of your chest.
19. Jump high 1 ½ stance distance; land in right cross-footed stance and perform a lower level X block. Kiai.
20. Step 90° to the right into a right inline forward stance and perform a right augmented block.
21. Pivot to the front into a left forward stance; perform a left upper level sweep block and a right lower level strike, then step into a left back stance while performing a left down block and a right upper level inside forearm block behind your head.
22. Withdraw your right front leg to the feet together position with your body facing to the right side.
23. Pivot on your left foot and step forward into a right forward stance while

performing a right upper level sweep block and a left lower level strike. Then step into a right back stance while performing a right down block and a left upper level inside forearm block behind your head.

Withdraw your right leg, return to natural stance and demonstrate zanshin – remaining mind. Move your left leg halfway towards your right leg, then your right leg halfway towards your left leg into the feet together, toes open stance, and bow.

The Tekki Katas

The purple belt kata is Tekki Shodan and is the first of 3 katas in the Tekki group. The Tekki katas move in a straight line from side to side and are primarily in side stance. The focus is on sharp head movements and strong quick body movements.

Tekki Shodan

Start from the feet together position, with your toes open, and bow. Bring your toes together and place your open left hand on top of your open right, palms facing towards your body at a 30-degree angle from your shoulders.

1. Keep your hands in their position and quickly cross your left foot over your right foot with the ball of your foot touching the floor and your heel off the ground. Turn your head sharply and look to the right.
2. Press your left heel onto the floor, raise your right knee up to chest height and stomp the ground with your right foot as you step into side stance. At the same time extend your right arm to the side and perform a backhand block while your left hand is pulled to the draw hand position at your hip.
3. Using body rotation, perform a left forward elbow strike to the right using your right open hand as a target.
4. Turn your head sharply to the left and stack your left fist on top of your right in the draw-hand position.
5. Using body vibration, down block with your left arm to the left side.
6. Perform a right middle body level hook punch to the left side.
7. Keep your arms in their positions, cross your right foot in front of your left foot placing the ball of the foot on the floor with your heel off the ground.
8. Press your right heel into the floor, raise your left knee up to chest height and stomp the ground with your left foot as you step into side stance. As your foot hits the floor turn your head sharply to the front and twist your right arm from the hook punch position to a middle level inside forearm block.
9. Bring your right arm up to your left shoulder in preparation for a down block while extending your left arm forward as though you were punching to the lower body. Perform a right down block while sweeping your left arm up to your left ear. Perform a right closed-fist pressing block while back-fist striking upper body with your left arm.
10. Leaving your arms in position turn your head sharply to the left.
11. Perform a left inside snap kick (wave kick) then rotate your hip sharply to the left and block with the outer surface of your left forearm using an inside forearm block motion.
12. Keep the same position and turn your head sharply to the right.
13. Perform a right inside snap kick (wave kick) then rotate your hip sharply to the right and block with the outer surface of your left forearm using an outside forearm block motion.
14. Turn your head sharply to the left and stack your left fist on top of your right in the draw-hand position.
15. Perform a left middle body punch-block and a right middle-body hook punch to the left. Kiai.
16. Open both hands, cross your left arm in front of your body under your right arm, and your right arm over your left arm, then perform a left vertical sword

hand block to the left and immediately change it into a back hand block.

17. Using body rotation, perform a right forward elbow strike to the left using your left open hand as a target.
18. Turn your head sharply to the right and stack your right fist on top of your left in the draw-hand position.
19. Using body vibration, down block with your right arm to the right side.
20. Perform a left middle body level hook punch to the right side.
21. Keep your arms in their positions, cross your left foot in front of your right foot placing the ball of the foot on the floor with your heel off the ground.
22. Press your left heel into the floor, raise your right knee up to chest height and stomp the ground with your right foot as you step into side stance. As your foot hits the floor turn your head sharply to the front and twist your left arm from the hook punch position to a middle level inside forearm block.
23. Bring your left arm up to your right shoulder in preparation for a down block while extending your right arm forward as though you were punching to the lower body. Perform a left down block while sweeping your right arm up to your right ear. Perform a left closed-fist pressing block while back-fist striking upper body with your right arm.
24. Leaving your arms in position turn your head sharply to the right.
25. Perform a right inside snap kick (wave kick) then rotate your hip sharply to the right and block with the outer surface of your right forearm using an inside forearm block motion.
26. Keep the same position and turn your head sharply to the left.
27. Perform a left inside snap kick (wave kick) then rotate your hip sharply to the left and block with the outer surface of your right forearm using an outside forearm block motion.
28. Turn your head sharply to the right and stack your right fist on top of your left in the draw-hand position.
29. Perform a right middle body punch-block and a left middle-body hook punch to the right. Kiai.

Return to the feet-together toes-open position by drawing your right foot over to your left foot. Open both hands and return to the starting position of the kata wherein both hands are positioned in front of your body with your left hand stacked on top of your right hand. Pause for a moment, demonstrate zanshin, open the toes and bow; then return to natural stance.

The Advanced Katas

Once you reach 3rd kyu brown belt you will learn the next five katas: Bassai Dai, Kanku Dai, Jion, Empi, and Tekki Nidan. One of these katas will be assigned to you according to your body type and personality. This is the kata that you will perform for your 2nd and 3rd kyu brown belt test and for your 1st degree black belt test. After you earn 1st degree black belt you will learn the katas Gankaku, Jutte, Hangetsu, as well as Tekki Sandan. The five Heian katas, the three Tekki katas, and Bassai Dai, Kanku Dai, Jion, Empi, Gankaku, Jutte, and Hangetsu make up the 15 core katas of Shotokan Karate. There are an additional 11 katas that complete the 26 katas of Shotokan Karate. Those katas are generally divided into two groups. The first group of five consists of Bassai Sho, Kanku Sho, Chinte, Sochin and Nijushiho. The second group of six consists of Unsu, Gojushiho Sho, Gojushiho Dai, Meikyo, Wankan and Ji'in.

Further explanation of these katas can be found in the <u>Best Karate</u> series, by Masatoshi Nakayama, and in various youtube videos. To find them go to youtube and type in the name of the kata you'd like to see. You should find several examples.

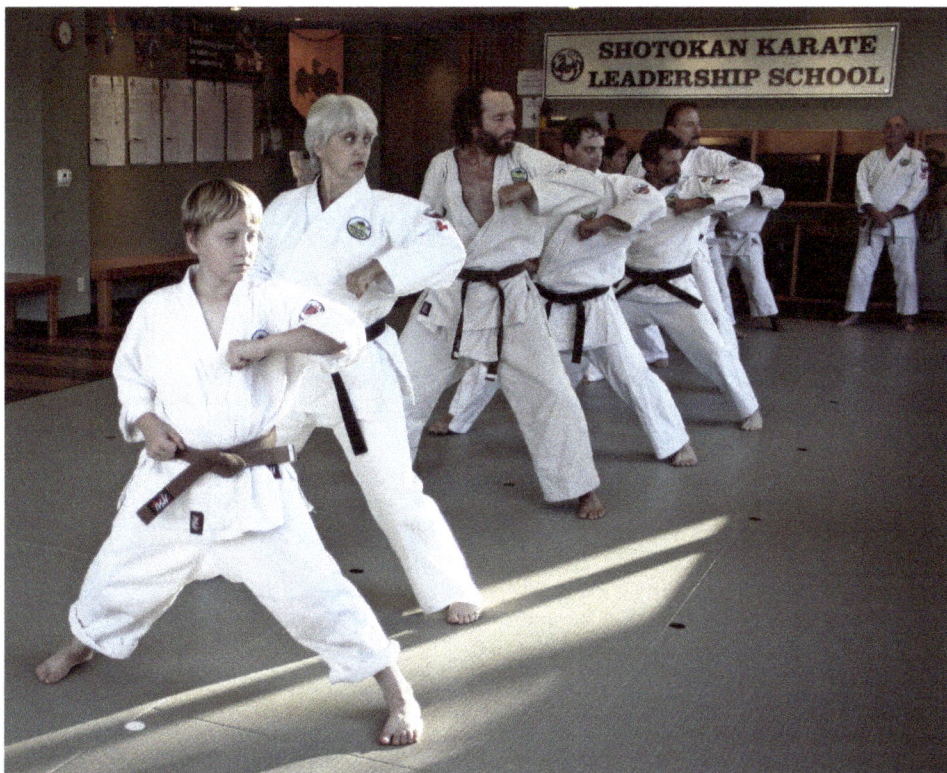

Conditioning Exercises

Do anywhere from 3 to 20 or more repetitions of each exercise

Crunches – 10 positions

We perform crunches from 10 different positions. Start by laying flat on your back with either your arms across your chest or with your hands touching your shoulders. Then sit up at approximately a 45° angle.

1. Knees bent, feet together and flat on the floor
2. Knees open, soles of the feet together and edges of the feet on the floor
3. Knees together, ankles crossed, feet off the floor
4. Knees open, soles of the feet together and off the floor
5. Legs straight, held tightly together, pointing straight up
6. Legs open in a big Y
7. Right leg straight about 6 inches off the floor, left leg bent close to the chest
8. Reverse: left leg straight about 6 inches off the floor, right leg bent close to the chest
9. Turn onto your right side and bend both knees close to your chest
10. Turn onto your left side and bend both knees close to your chest

Leg raises – 2 positions

1. Lying on your right side, bend your right knee, keep your left leg straight and raise it straight up
2. Repeat but with the left bent
3. Repeat on other side

Back arches – 2 positions

1. Lay flat on your stomach with your arms extended out in front, arch your head/shoulders and your legs up.
2. Lay flat on your stomach with your arms down to your sides, arch your head/shoulders and your legs up.

Knuckle pushups

Lie flat on your stomach and place your closed fists next to the draw hand position with the thumb side of your fist towards your head. Push up to a straight-arm position then lower yourself down close to the floor. Alternatively push up to a half-straight arm position then lower yourself down close to the floor. And, starting with your arms straight lower yourself down part way to the floor and return to the straight arm position.

Squat kicks

From the natural stance position open your feet just enough so that when you squat down both of your heels remain on the floor. Stand up, front-snap kick with your right leg and squat down again. Stand up again and front-snap kick with your left leg and squat down.

Repeat multiple times.

Breathing exercises

Stand in a wide natural stance with your arms down and your hands touching. Take a deep breath in and raise your arms up to a position high above your head. Breathe out slowly and circle your arms down and around returning your arms to the lower position. Take another deep breath in and raise your arms straight out to your sides at shoulder height. Breathe out slowly and lower your arms down to the position in front of your body.

Repeat this sequence once more.

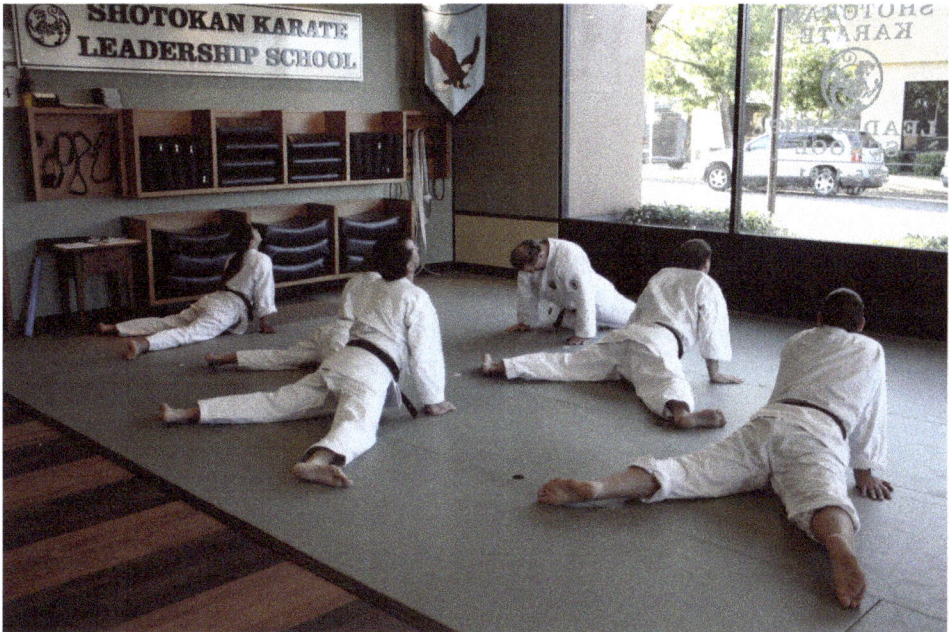

Appendix

Japanese Terminology

Numbers

ICHI: one
NI: two
SAN: three
SHI: four
GO: five

ROKU: six
SHICHI: seven
HACHI: eight
KU: nine
JU: ten

General Terms

CHUDAN: middle body
DAN: black belt ranks
DOJO: training hall
GEDAN: lower body
GI: karate uniform
HAJIME: begin
JODAN: upper body
KAMAE: ready position
KIAI: shout or yell
KYU: belt levels below black belt
MOKUSO: meditation
OSU: yes, exclamation of spirit
REI: bow
SENSEI: one who has gone before, teacher
SHOMEN: front
YAME: stop

Techniques

Stances

FUDO (SOCHIN) DACHI: rooted stance
HANGETSU DACHI: wide hourglass stance
KIBA DACHI: side stance
KOKUTSU DACHI: back stance
KOSA DACHI: crossed feet stance
NEKO ASHI DACHI: cat-legged stance
SANCHIN DACHI: hourglass stance
SHIZEN TAI: natural stance
ZENKUTSU DACHI: forward stance

Kicking

MAE KEAGE GERI: front snap kick
MAE KEKOMI GERI: front thrust kick
MAWASHI GERI: round house kick
USHIRO KEKOMI GERI: back thrust kick
YOKO KEAGE GERI: side snap kick
YOKO KEKOMI GERI: side thrust kick

Punching

GYAKU ZUKI: reverse punch
KIZAMI ZUKI: short punch
OI ZUKI : step-in punch
TSUKI : straight punch

Blocking

AGE UKE : rising block
GEDAN BARAI : down block
MOROTE UKE: augmented block
SHUTO UKE: sword hand block
SOTO UKE: outside forearm block
UCHI UKE: inside forearm block

Striking

EMPI UCHI: elbow strike
SHUTO UCKI : sword hand strike
URAKEN: back fist strike

Ranking System

The ranking system is broken into three divisions. Belt stripes for very young children ages 3 to 6. *Kyu* (pronounced "cue") for ranks below black belt, and *dan* (pronounced "dahn") for black belt ranks.

There are four stripes for ages 3 to 6.

1. Bear Stripe for stances and body positions
2. Eagle Stripe for upper body techniques
3. Fire Dragon Stripe for lower body techniques
4. Kraken Stripe for moving from stance to stance and turning.

Kyu Ranks

Unranked – White Belt
11th Kyu – White Belt with Yellow Stripe
10th Kyu – White Belt with Orange Stripe
9th Kyu – White Belt with Green Stripe
8th Kyu – Yellow Belt
7th Kyu – Orange Belt
6th Kyu – Green Belt
5th Kyu – Blue Belt
4th Kyu – Purple Belt
3rd Kyu – Brown Belt
2nd Kyu – Brown Belt
1st Kyu – Brown Belt

Dan Ranks

1st Dan – Shodan
2nd Dan – Nidan
3rd Dan – Sandan
4th Dan – Yondan
5th Dan – Godan
6th Dan – Rokudan
7th Dan – Shichidan
8th Dan – Hachidan
9th Dan – Kudan
10th Dan – Judan

YouTube

Shotokan Karate Leadership School® has a YouTube account where you can view students demonstrating the correct way to do a kata or the proper way to bow. Check out our channel at www.youtube.com/channels/shotokankarateleadershipschool.

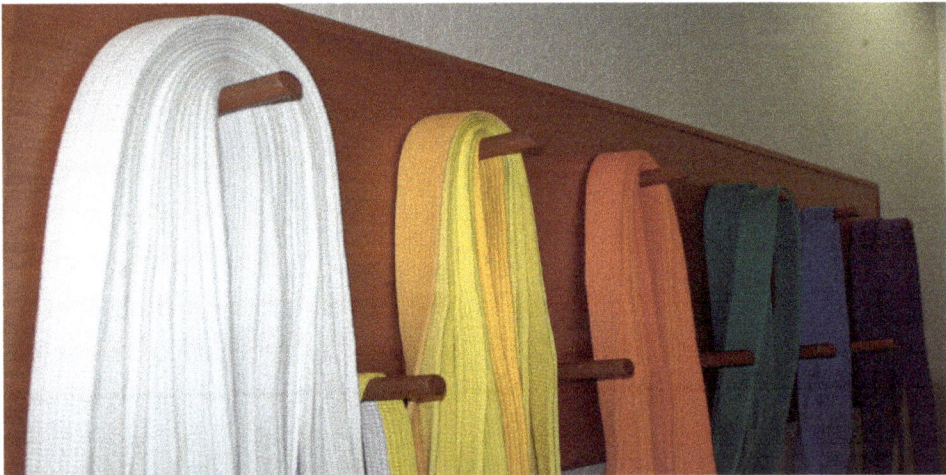

This Shoka Leader Handbook

Belongs to: _____

Date I Became A:

11th kyu White Yellow Stripe_____

10th kyu White Orange Stripe_____

9th kyu White Green Stripe_____

8th kyu Yellow Belt _____

7th kyu Orange Belt _____

6th kyu Green Belt _____

5th kyu Blue Belt _____

4th kyu Purple Belt _____

3rd kyu Brown Belt _____

2nd kyu Brown Belt _____

1st kyu Brown Belt _____

1st dan Black Belt _____

2nd dan Black Belt _____

3rd dan Black Belt_____

4th dan Black Belt_____

5th dan Black Belt_____

Class Leader _____

House Leader _____

School Leader _____

Assistant Instructor _____

Junior Instructor _____

Instructor _____

Praise for Shotokan Karate Leadership School
& Sensei Marty Callahan

*"Sensei, my name is Dean. I was your student 15 years ago. I'm calling because I want to thank you for giving me the **foundation for a wonderful life**. The training I received from you has helped me in innumerable ways. I have a **wonderful life** and I don't believe it would have turned out this way without the training that I received from you. Thank you from the bottom of my heart."*

-Dean, June of 2011

*"I'm not sure you remember me, but my name is Benjamin Wright son of who is now Marta May. I was instructed in Shotokan in my early years at your dojo on Hall Road. I wanted to contact you and thank you for your instruction. You taught me **discipline and honor**, which have given me an advantage when interacting with my peers. I cannot find the words to describe the attributes I have developed from your lessons, but these attributes give me confidence as I prepare to leave for college."*

-Benjamin Wright

"My son Braden's confidence and interpersonal skills have changed tremendously over the past year. SKLS has played a crucial role in the improvement we have seen. Thank you, Sensei, for your attention to detail and the guidance that you have given my son."

-Kirsten, February 2010

"My son, Jared, trained with you about 25 years ago when he was 8 years old. We enrolled him in your school because he was being bullied at school. He left feeling much more confident and went on to become a physician. He now practices medicine in Portland Oregon. We are very grateful for what you did."

-Janice Shipley, Feb. 4, 2012